Solitary

Tyler Coburn

I went to Korea to put myself in prison.

This may sound a bit misleading, so let me start again.

In 2013, a facility was built in the hills of Hongcheon, about an hour east of Seoul. On almost every side is a clear view of forest.

The facility is run by an organization called Happitory—a combination of "Happiness" and "Factory." Happitory caters to people who want to disengage from their busy daily lives and reengage themselves. To this end, a total of 28 guests can check into its building, which is designed like a prison. Happitory offers retreats for teenagers, company employees, government officials, and the general public. Some sessions involve drama therapy, others are led by Buddhist monks. Most intriguing is a program of "solitary confinement," where one can spend twenty-four hours of technology-free time locked in an individual cell.

I learned about Happitory when it opened; in July 2019, I finally had an opportunity to visit. In the pages that follow, I will share some associations and reflections from my "solitary confinement," then introduce the contributions to this book.

*

Central to Happitory's philosophy is "Prison Inside Me": the belief that we all live within restrictions. Some are self-imposed, others are not. Many become habit and scarcely register in our conscious thought. Inside such strictures, we build a life; to these tight bindings, we accommodate ourselves.

Seen through this lens, Happitory's mock prison appears less like an exceptional space—less like an oddity in the relaxation-industrial complex. Indeed, we don't enter "prison" when we arrive at Happitory: we recognize, possibly for the first time, that we are already jailed. For the duration of our stay, we live inside ourselves living inside a concretized version of ourselves. We are doubly imprisoned, trapped in a redundancy.

Perhaps, when a metaphor is this strained, it collapses under its weight. Perhaps, by overdetermining prison, we can finally feel free.

*

Freedom through restriction. It's something many people I know seek out in their leisure time. I think of the silent retreat, which my father has done several times in middle age. As the days progress, he recently told me, his thoughts become slower and slower as if, freed from the work of transforming into speech, they could take a more comfortable pace.

I think of the sensory deprivation tank, the anechoic chamber. There's a famous story about John Cage visiting such a chamber at Harvard. Surely this would be the world's quietest place—where silence might make itself known. Yet even inside the chamber, there was noise: the pulsations of Cage's nervous system, the rush of blood through his veins and arteries. These sounds accompany us throughout our lives but are dampened by the din of the world. Finally, they could be heard.

Reflecting on his experience, Cage wrote: "Until I die there will be sounds. And they will continue following my death. One need not fear about the future of music."[1]

*

By restricting ourselves, we free ourselves. A higher plane of awareness is reached. This trope appears in many cultures often embodied by the figure of the blind, who loses an eye on the material world and gains a view of the divine.

Being so reliant on sight, as philosophers like to remind, we risk becoming trapped in the realm of appearances, taking what is evident to the eyes as tantamount to truth. For the blind, does another sense assume the predominance of vision, or do they all share the spoils? I don't know, but I like something Diderot has written: in blindness, the skin becomes a giant canvas upon which the world figures itself.[2]

Borges became blind in later life—ironically, around the time he assumed the directorship of the National Library in Buenos Aires. So many books, and barely a pair of eyes to read them! In writing about his condition, Borges dispels the common conception of blindness as darkness. The blind don't peer into the void, he argues, so much as through a "greenish or blueish mist, vaguely luminous."[3] Living in the shadow of the visual world, colors and effects persist.

*

A few weeks before my stay at Happitory, I read Jun'ichirō Tanizaki's *In Praise of Shadows* on the recommendation of my boyfriend. I was surprised by the tone of the text. Given its title, I expected a spare meditation on Japanese aesthetics, not a snarky piece of design commentary that opens with several pages devoted to the toilet. Tanizaki's taste leans traditional and often outside his budget. His perfect bathroom would include a wooden urinal "filled with boughs of cedar," its fixtures finished in "glistening black lacquer."[4] To eat food under electric light is effectively to destroy it.

The title of Tanizaki's book comes from his discussion of the home. Whereas the Western home is built with a small roof and glass windows to let in as much light as possible, the Japanese home lacks glass so needs a roof, sized like a parasol, to keep out rain and wind. In such a home, shadows collect. They patina the alcoves and corners, as if fleshing out hollowed skins—forming a "quality of mystery and depth," he writes, "superior to that of any wall painting or ornament."[5]

*

My boyfriend visited me in Korea, and on our first afternoon together, we went to Gyeonghuigung Palace. The palace, like several others in Seoul, is a composite that appears to be a seamless whole. Burned, dismantled—torn asunder—it has been partially made anew. A plaque installed on the site traces its greatest damage to the period between 1910 and 1945. If one could read the seamlines, they'd tell a story of colonialism.

As we walked around the palace grounds, I told my boyfriend that I had finished *In Praise of Shadows*, expecting to earn some points. He sheepishly confessed that he had never actually read it.

I'll admit, I was shocked. I guess I had assumed that, in recommending the book, he was offering a window onto his youth in Japan—and his particular aesthetic sensibility. How would I describe that sensibility? Well, once, when we were walking through Donald Judd's former SoHo apartment, we came upon a thin, threadbare mat where the sculptor would take his naps. (I watched my boyfriend make a mental note.) In the home he imagines we'll eventually share, there will be a single large table: for eating, working, and fucking.

*

One week before my boyfriend came to Korea, I read *Escape to Prison*, a 2015 book about prison tourism. As part of his fieldwork, author Michael Welch visited the Seodaemun Prison History Hall, a museum built into the most notorious jail of the Japanese colonial era. Its displays include mugshots, artifacts, and the extremely unusual "Shadow Image Experiment," where a visitor can have their body scanned as a silhouette, which is then embedded in a video on a nearby screen. Over the next ninety seconds, the silhouette undergoes incarceration, interrogation, and torture at the hands of animated Japanese officers. One becomes familiar with the atrocities committed in this place by seeing one's very own shadow suffer.

Two weeks after my boyfriend left Korea, I visited the Seodaemun Prison History Hall to experience the "Shadow Image Experiment" myself, but in its place, I found a video marking the 100th anniversary of the March First Independence Movement. A wall text encouraged visitors, as they watched, to shout "Long Live Korea!"

*

I know: I'm digressing. I should write about my time in a happiness factory designed as a prison.

Certainly, there are things to share. Three times a day, a tidy Tupperware meal arrived outside my door, which I could collect through a slot. At 9:30pm, I heard an officer checking the locks.

In the hours that followed, the facility approached a painful degree of silence, interrupted only once by a Kakao sound—evidence of a contraband smartphone.

Morning began at 6am with a soothing tone played through a ceiling speaker. A woman's voice, run through the mill of postproduction echo effects, guided me in meditation. She finished, and I fell back asleep. When I awoke again, I wasn't certain if I had heard her voice or dreamt it.

Little can be brought into the cell. Toiletries and pajamas are allowed, but no electronics—and usually no books. "Every person is a book," an officer remarked, suggesting that one will have all the reading material needed to pass the twenty-four hours.

Inside my cell I found bedding, a yoga mat, an electric kettle, and a tea set. On a small table sat a pack of markers, a notebook, a notepad, and envelopes.

The notebook contained reflections by past residents of my cell. The notepad could be used for letters: to family, friends, even oneself. Happitory's officers will collect sealed envelopes and ensure they reach their intended destinations.

*

By providing these supplies (whether intentionally or not) Happitory taps into the history of prison writing, following in the footsteps of as varied a group as Oscar Wilde, Antonio Gramsci, and Shin Young-bok.

For many, writing materials weren't readily available. The Reverend Martin Luther King Jr. penned his 1963 "Letter from Birmingham Jail" in the margins and between the ads of the newspaper, on any paper towels and napkins he could find. King's lawyer and speechwriter would visit him twice a day, stashing the scraps between the buttonholes of his shirt.

In 2013, Behrouz Boochani fled a journalistic crackdown in Iran, only to find himself indefinitely detained on Manus Island. Fearful that his writing paper would be searched and seized, he typed his memoir over a series of WhatsApp messages to his translator. It's bitterly ironic that, though Boochani was unable to enter Australia, the memoir, *No Friend But the Mountains*, won the country's 2019 Victorian Prize for Literature.

He was granted refugee status by New Zealand the following year.

*

Kim Dae-jung once famously remarked, “I wish I could go back to prison,” yearning for the time it afforded to read and write.[6] Freedom through restriction: there’s that theme again. It was only when imprisoned that Marco Polo stopped and told the story of his travels to an inmate who happened to be a writer—only then that the Marquis de Sade experienced his most prolific periods. (It’s worth mentioning that Sade spent more than a third of his life behind bars.)

Prison is even a template for writers who never went to jail. Annie Dillard found the view through her office window so distracting that she moved her desk to face a blank wall. “Appealing workplaces are to be avoided,” she reflects. “One wants a room with no view, so imagination can meet memory in the dark.”[7]

*

I lied to you earlier when I apologized for digressing. I wasn’t sorry, and in fact, I hadn’t digressed at all. Most of what you’ve read was drafted during my period of “solitary confinement.” The blind, the shadow, my boyfriend are facets of the experience—thoughts that passed the time.

It would be reckless to call this writing process “liberating,” or claim that my confinement felt freeing, as so little of my experience approximated that of an actual prisoner. I chose to enter Happitory's "prison." I had the privilege of leaving at any time by pressing a panic button in my room.

This is not to say that I doubt the sincerity of the facility's founders. One of them, Jihyang Noh, has done drama therapy with inmates and other marginalized communities for much of her working life. Noh told me that the prison system can only do so much; rehabilitation requires more than time in jail. As a testament to this belief, she's been leading sessions at Happitory for juvenile offenders and their families—a wrenching attempt to look beyond the symptoms.

*

When Happitory opened in 2013, the main program it offered was "Prison Inside Me," but the founders came to realize that the name scared off potential clients. "Prison Inside Me" was thus rebranded with terms like "Happy Reflection," softening a metaphor still unavoidable in the facility's architecture.

Shortly after the imprisonment of Park Geun-hye,[8] Happitory reintroduced the word "prison" with a new program: "Twenty Hours in Prison to Change Ourselves and Our Society." The timing expressed the urgency—even for a wellness center—of reflecting on the state of the country and its elected leaders. To what extent, the title seems to ask, is her guilt our own? Have we become complacent about the political status quo?

I don't mean to include myself in this "we." Though

Happitory has received a fair amount of Western press, its website is only in Korean so doesn't actively target foreigners. Nor can I appreciate the nuance of how it operates within the Korean imaginary. To fully engage this facility, I needed to bring in other voices. I imagined turning the mock prison into a writing residency…

*

Since my stay, I've arranged for nine colleagues based in Korea to visit Happitory. I invited them to produce writing on site, like I did, bringing their interests and life stories to bear on the experience of "solitary confinement." Their texts fill the rest of this book.

Kyungmook Kim was once imprisoned for being a conscientious objector to military service; he spent approximately fifteen months of his sentence in solitary confinement. Kyungmook reflects on that period from his room in Happitory's simulation, describing the "repressive order" of the carceral regime and the "imaginary spaces" he had to build as a means of survival. The virtual world, Kyungmook observes, is "an ancient, intrinsic characteristic of humans that can be created without any technology."

As a member of Yellow Pen Club, Jiwon Yu has run alternative writing workshops that hone participants' observational techniques—and which resonate with the experimental premise of this book. In her text, Jiwon finds similarities between Happitory and the retreats that Korean youth attend: "[t]here is something particularly liberating" in the way they remove "the mundane responsibilities of life." Jiwon was the second contributor to visit the facility, in February 2020; the pandemic plays a role in her text.

Woochang Lee's essay, "Prison, Solitude, and the 'True Self,'" provides a framework for comparing the self-care promoted by Happitory to the philosophical tradition of the "care of the self." Woochang traces conceptions of freedom, solitude, discipline, and selfhood through western thought as well as modern Korean history, addressing the importance of prison letters in the country's democratization movement.

The chance discovery of some coins in Sunjin Kim's pocket gave the author an idea: to summon "the ancient wisdom of the *Book of Changes* from inside a cell where one can't sense any change." Sunjin's text unfolds in questions posed to the oracle about NFTs, electric cars, food insecurity—the subjects of our time. He takes some creative license with his experience at Happitory, making the staff seem hostile for dramatic effect.

To pass the hours in her room, Jaeyeon Chung kept singing *Nostalgia*, a song based on a poem by Jeong Jiyong that she learned in middle school. Jaeyeon could recall the melody, though the lyrics were "blurry," the words "wandering about." As she tries to remember them, her text becomes a portrait of the act of memory, dotted with ellipses. Jaeyeon had wanted to spend this time meditating but couldn't quiet her active mind.

In a nearby room, Jaeyeon's husband Russell Mason was also struggling to meditate, distracted by the need to write something for this book. What results is a text-within-a-text: a treatise on the limits of knowing the world, and the story of writing that treatise. When complete, Russell jokes that he has "almost settled the issues plaguing the western mind for centuries." He returns to meditation and feels a true sense of gratitude.

InYoung Yeo told me that she interprets the world "in numbers, dimensions, and patterns." Within her room at Happitory, she trained her focus on the walls, windows, ceilings, and light fixtures—watching them extend "into the spaces above, below, and all around." InYoung's text is a record of this experience as well as a theoretical proposition, exploring what "new sensibilities" might exist in "the ternary relationship among human, nature, and technology."[9]

When Hyunjeung Kim visited Happitory in January 2021, she was at work on an exhibition at Gyeonggi Museum of Modern Art, in Ansan, that commemorates the seventh anniversary of the Sewol ferry disaster. In her text, Hyunjeung discusses the forms of digital solidarity that emerged in its wake. She also reflects on the disaster within the context of the pandemic, wondering about "the role of art in the time of catastrophe—and for those in need of consolation."

Min Kyoung Lee once conducted an experiment in "radical ethnology": she would stay in a monastery until she gained enlightenment, then return "to the secular world and report it in an artistic product."[10] The risk, she acknowledged, was that she might never leave, converting from artist to seeker. Min came back to us then, but in her text, she's again seeking enlightenment. As Happitory appropriates aspects of monastic life, perhaps she will find it there?

Taken as a whole, *Solitary* is a unique publication in being both a collection of texts and a collective work, which explores the possibilities of site-specific writing. It is indebted to the discourses of critical spatial practice and site-specific art—particularly, to Miwon Kwon's claim that a site can be physical, institutional, and discursive. Happitory exists at the nexus of the three, extruding carceral tropes into physical and institutional forms. How, we ten contributors ask, can one capture this site through embedded, embodied writing? What stories does Happitory have to tell about solitude and introspection, punishment and repair?

1. John Cage, *Silence: Lectures and Writings* (Middletown, CT: Wesleyan University Press, 1961).

2. See Diderot's "Letter on the Blind for the Use of Those Who Can See" (1749).

3. Jorge Luis Borges, "Blindness" (1977).

4. Jun'ichirō Tanizaki, *In Praise of Shadows* (1933; Sedgwick, ME: Leete's Island Books, 1977).

5. Ibid.

6. Kim Dae-jung (1924–2009) served as President of South Korea from 1998 to 2003. He was the first liberal leader elected to this position. In his earlier life, Kim was a notable dissident sentenced to death in 1980; the sentence was commuted to a twenty-year prison term, and that term was suspended in 1982, when Kim went into exile in the United States until 1985. Woochang Lee discusses Kim's prison writings in his contribution to this book.

7. Annie Dillard, *The Writing Life* (New York: HarperCollins Publishers, 1989).

8. Park Geun-hye served as President of South Korea from 2013 to 2017. She was impeached on corruption charges and sentenced to twenty-four years in prison.

9. These quotes come from an email exchange with InYoung in April 2021.

10. Min Kyoung Lee, *Art, as Necessary* (2016).

Kyungmook Kim

A mind going
To the sky to the sky
If you ride
Clear wind
White clouds
Will wash your tears

— Kim Kwang-seob, *Leaning on the Prison Window*

Imprisonment

As a conscientious objector to military service, I spent about fifteen months in solitary confinement at the Nambu and Tongyeong detention centers from January 2015 to March 2016. Through Happitory's program, I again experienced solitary—four years later.

Like most prison facilities, Happitory is located on the outskirts of the city, far from society. The admission procedure is similar as well. Upon entering, I changed into a uniform and received a name tag with my room number written on it. I'm not sure if it was intended, but the color of the uniform was similar to that of actual prison clothes, and the room number on the name tag reminded me of the ones inmates are given. This intake process is a significant ritual act, which forms one's identity as a prisoner: I am no longer in society but belong to the correctional facility.

Room 203, where I stayed at Happitory, was not so unfamiliar. Measuring five meters square, it had a door that could not be unlocked from the inside; a slot to distribute food; a cramped bathroom and basin; a palm-sized mirror above the toilet; a small trash can; and a floor desk. There were other similarities: you go to bed at 10pm and wake up at 6am, you cannot leave the room until the end of the program. All you can do in the meantime are individual activities like reading and writing.

The first things I did when I entered the room were yoga and meditation: how I used to start my day in prison. These practices trained me to endure that period in sound mind—without going crazy. By repeating it at Happitory, I regained a sense of how to breathe and move in confined space. I prepared to meet a former version of myself who was also a prisoner. Memories and past selves dwell in space. Certain gestures and behaviors summon them.

The Solitary Room of Two Different Worlds

A solitary room in prison is more than a restricted space of 5.25 m^2. It is part of the carceral system: an institutional form of punishment with the legal force to suppress freedom. In this way, it differs from the solitary room at Happitory, which seeks to foster greater freedom by limiting one's freedom. Although the organization of the day is the same, waking up at 6am in prison is an obligation, not an option. If you do not wake up at that time, you will be punished. You also cannot lie down in the room apart from bedtime, and you cannot take off your prison uniform even in the heat of summer. It is prohibited to exercise in the room, use a towel as a cushion, or stand without reason. These rules must be followed from the moment you enter prison. Otherwise, punishment ensues.

Prison is a world of repressive order, where discipline and obedience are the top priorities. Although I was able to adapt to my narrow room, I could not get used to a system built on subordination. It was difficult for me to sit for a long time, due to back pain, so the lack of any chair or cushion worsened my health. However, compared to other prisoners suffering severe physical consequences from long sentences, my case was pretty manageable.

The window in room 203 occupied much of a wall, showing a delicate scene stitched with trees. The window in my former solitary cell was small; through it, I could only see another wall of the same building. While the walls of that prison were faded gray, this place is a white cube just like an art gallery.

That said, the experience provided by Happitory isn't completely different from the one I had in prison. Both institutions emphasize self-discipline and create meditative spaces that are adequate for self-reflection. Happitory does so by romanticizing incarceration, with its quiet and peaceful rooms. In prison, self-discipline and self-reflection are only possible within a system of oppression and surveillance.

Space of Spirit

A solitary room, by its nature, leads to a deep interior life. If you stay in this room for long enough, you will fall into a meditative state, where the body remains in physical space, and the mind resides on a spiritual plane.

While living in solitary confinement, I tried to find freedom through my own virtual world. Although stuck in a tiny room for fifteen months, I was able to occupy imaginary spaces through letters from friends, books, meditation, and dreams. I could only breathe freely in this world I created for myself. Whenever I felt oppressed by prison life, I became more dependent on it: a way of surviving the physical restriction, which was close to violence. Over this period, I came to realize that the virtual world is not a specific place, like the internet, but an ancient, intrinsic characteristic of humans that can be created without any technology.

The room at Happitory is designed to help those who are tired of social life and human relationships focus on personal reflection and healing. It is also a digital detox program, requiring that participants spend time without their devices—apart from the hyper-connected, around-the-clock world. In room 203, there's a guestbook with entries by past occupants, some of whom were experiencing digital burnout. An excerpt on the following page claims that taking care of oneself means blocking out the surrounding world. This reminds me of when I lived in mind and memory—when I went inside myself, denying the existence of the cell that contained me and the prison around it, so nothing could hurt me.

When I can't sleep
I imagine that
I trapped myself somewhere
I am trapped in the space
Where no one can hurt me
Where no one can find me
Where time is stopped
And I can go out whenever I recover
This space has the same condition symbolically
Perhaps that's why I can fall asleep here

Isn't "Prison Inside Me" a symbolic realization
Of this kind of place
Where I can always hide?
You are not here because you have sinned,
But you came here
To protect yourself

Among the people who left traces in the guestbook were adults and many teenagers as well, staying at Happitory on school or club outings. They explained why they came here and the impressions they felt in the room. What interested me was how the writing of the adults and teenagers differed. Those of my generation and older wrote self-reflective inner monologues: the guestbook functioned as a diary. Teenagers' texts, by contrast, were directed to the people who would later read them—implicitly, members of their generation. Instagram handles were left. Entries ended with sentences like "Let's get to know each other by sharing more stories through Instagram DM." Writing in the guestbook was continuous with their digital lives—and actively mediated by the existence of others.

Night and Day

Around 7:50pm, the sun went down, and the sky began to darken. When I first entered the room, it was raining, but that stopped by now. I had wanted to meditate during the rain while gazing at the picturesque landscape. Instead, I listened to the crickets, frogs, and chirping birds; the humid atmosphere caused a reverb effect. I became tranquil, drunk on the sounds of the forest. I couldn't sleep even after bedtime, so I started to read *Reflections from Prison*, a 1988 book by Shin Young-Bok. "Today is just the day I wait for tomorrow. Today is yesterday's tomorrow, and tomorrow is just tomorrow's today." This sentence, which I repeated hundreds of times when I was imprisoned, still broke my heart. Shin was incarcerated in 1969 as an ideological prisoner and prisoner of conscience. He spent twenty years behind bars until being released on special parole on August 15, 1988. I remember how devastated I was after hearing his obituary in 2016, while I was still serving time. When I opened the book again, it felt as if he was still in prison. His body was laid to rest, but his mind will live forever in the letters he left behind.

At 6am the next morning, a calm ringtone woke me up. It was the soundtrack of the movie *My Neighbor Totoro* played with a music box. I could hear the birds, water, and wind outside my window; the sound of the world waking up is beautiful. At the same time, I felt keenly how much this place was unlike my former prison cell, where I woke up to the propaganda music of the Ministry of Justice: "The more I follow the law, the better I feel." Room 203 didn't give me stress or anxiety but offered time to soak up some peace and tranquility. The exterior of the building looked like a real prison, but there was no repressive discipline. If I remove the physical and mental punishment of prison and leave only the ideal aspects, like meditative self-reflection, then it becomes a solitary room at Happitory.

No one who participates in this program should feel they're in a real prison. As you can see in the program name, what you find here is a "Prison Inside Me": a place to learn that we are living in a prison called society. Happitory teaches us that prison is the world outside this room.

Jiwon Yu

1.

"You're not coming from Daegu, are you?"

She asked with a welcoming smile. On my way to Hongcheon, I was bombarded by the latest news about the spike of confirmed cases in Daegu. Right before I turned in my phone, I checked: 364 in total. I wondered if I had made the right decision to travel.

Hongcheon station was nearly empty, which might explain why my taxi driver was relieved to see me. When we reached Happitory, he gave me his card, embarrassed but insistent that I call him when I plan to return.

It was a surprise to find nearly a dozen other guests at Happitory, looking for some peace of mind. As I changed into the uniform, I wondered for a moment whether I had the virus, and what that would mean. What if I unknowingly spread it to everyone here—or contract it and go back to work in Seoul? Would the museum shut down because of me? ~~Would I be *that* annoying assistant curator who traveled and ends up closing down the museum?~~ I was suddenly struck by the fact that we are, before anything else, a body: a potential host for the virus. To distance yourself is to care for others, and to refrain from encounters is an act of selflessness. Once you test positive, you are immediately reduced to a number. Information about your whereabouts joins the database, available to view on the grounds of public interest. You will be quarantined, unable to get past the door while, as a number, you will be omnipresent.

Things weren't this bad only a few weeks ago. People used to joke about how they wanted to test positive or cross paths with those who had, so they could get two weeks off and finally take a breather. Now, one dare not joke about such a thing, yet here I am entering voluntary quarantine. The "prison" of Happitory is like a twisted punchline.

2.

"Escaping the prison inside me"

So says the cover of the booklet they give me. I thought this was supposed to be a prison experience, but the staff have the most Zen faces, say all the right words, walk us through the freshest air, and feed us wholesome food. ~~All I wanted was to be locked up in my cell, but the orientation took longer than expected.~~ I was not prepared to reciprocate the friendly gestures nor share my reasons for being here, smiling and looking eager to participate, which I tried my best to do. The minute the door locked, I felt a surge of fatigue. There was also some pressure: the hours to come should be so inspiring that they'd change my life. ~~This is mostly thanks to the video they showed in the orientation.~~ It doesn't help that there's a crew reporting on this place; some foreign press sent a guy to spend the day in a cell. They asked for our understanding, with a promise that we won't be disturbed. We'll see.

~~I feel so bad leaving my husband and cats behind in the chaos of our apartment, after moving only two days ago. I hope they don't hate me too much for this.~~ I rarely get to enjoy the luxury of disappearing altogether. I've worked as a freelance everything for long enough to understand that being available is the key to good business. I was told that celebrities spend an exorbitant amount of money to keep up their looks and style even when they aren't doing much, spending just to *be*. Freelance workers pay a similar price, pretending they're unbreakable under pressure and reliable as a rock. They buffer themselves to manage precarity and insecurity, lest they fall off the map.

If the set of principles an individual imposes on herself is a *small system*, the social structures that necessitate it are the *big system*. This cell, for example, enforces a big system (albeit a temporary one) that fights off the preexisting big system so one's small system can get a chance to regroup. Growing up in Korea means entering at least one temporary big system every year, in the form of camps and retreats. To follow their protocols, you must forgo your digital devices; favorite clothes and accessories; and finally, your agency. These experiences accustom us to something we seek, in later life, through all sorts of masochistic fantasies: from mandatory new-recruit orientations to religious camps and meditation retreats, which promise to make a whole new person out of you. There is something particularly liberating about systems that eliminate or keep at bay the mundane responsibilities of life.

In my teens, I dreamed of being an independent woman. Then I spent all my twenties, independent as I so wanted, burdened with the task of self-organization in the face of countless variables—wishing I could be cornered and forced to abandon my obligations. Well, look where I am right now.

3.

In this compact room, there was nothing for me to do: no phone to hold for my sense of security, no laptop to be tapping on, not even a book to distract me. I shed all my extensions at the door, as was nicely but firmly requested. I managed to write quite a bit, to my surprise, then began to feel drowsy. I spread the quilt and lay down. It was the middle of the day, and I was rather excited about taking a nap.

I was pulling the blanket up to my face when I sensed something. I looked over at the door. Through a slit I saw a camera—a big one that belonged to the foreign press. I thought they promised not to bother us. Do they think it's fine as long as they aren't barging in? ~~He's still there even though I'm looking squarely at the camera. Should I throw something? Would that make me look crazy?~~ I thought of filing an official complaint then and there, but that's such an ordeal. I leaned into the corner so I wouldn't be in the shot.

~~I can't stop playing this new K-pop song in my head. What is wrong with me?~~

~~Fiesta! My heart swallowed the sun~~
~~In all seasons I will not wane, burning eternally~~
~~All is my season, every day a festival~~
~~Come to my fiesta someday...~~

4.

How long was I out?

I should have brought a watch. My phone swallowed my need for one, making the meaning of *clockwise* irrelevant. As I can't have it in the cell, there's no chance to watch the time tick by. There seems to be a bell ringing every hour, but it's no good. ~~It's so hard to count the number of rings.~~ I sleep then wake up, only to fall asleep again in this timeless void. It's pointless to bite myself and try to be efficient, when my sense of time is completely displaced. I don't have emails or calls to answer—not that I know of anyways. I'm getting drowsier by the minute and can't think of what to write. ~~Am I sleepy because of boredom?~~

Ever since I got my first smartphone, I've had earphones on all the time, except for when I simply must put them down. I hate to face what the world actually sounds like, so I put on loud music. I wish a humdrum afternoon to pass by listening to podcasts.

In a way, exposing myself to sound is a form of consumption, even when I'm not actually paying for it. The currency is my auditory attention. The act of streaming content delivers automatic feedback to the platform; that content is marketable, yielding ad cents for the creator.

Consumption tells a lot about a person: you are, not entirely but to a substantial extent, what you buy with your time. This room is completely silent. That means I'm not a consumer of any kind. In and out of sleep, I am only a body without a personality. I don't hate this. Not at all.

5.

~~How many times I've been in and out of sleep, I have not the slightest idea.~~
~~No can do a full sentence, no way.~~
~~Should have brought my journal to make things easier.~~
~~I hate this paper.~~
~~This isn't your journal, get it together. Don't be listing tacky epigrams, or am I already doing that?~~

Since I was little, I have kept a hand-written journal. Thoughts are almost always swifter than my hands, which learned the habit of writing concentrated impressions and expressions of emotion while leaving out factual details. This approach can make me quite vulnerable, exposing my prejudice and vice. I'm inclined to censor myself. Even in the privacy of a journal, the possibility of being read lurks...

With the exception of my journal, I usually write with a whole bunch of equipment: a monitor, keyboard, word processor, and more. It's almost impossible to go without online dictionaries and thesauruses, which make it much easier to toy around with words and find the perfect fit. My reliance on the internet is not due to my lack of basic knowledge of orthography, or so I'd like to believe. I've come to consider the search bar a part of my writing brain, and cloud storage an extension of my memory. Writing without them simply feels wrong, as if I'm not quite myself, struggling to form a sentence, let alone structure a paragraph. My first readers, usually the editor or dear friends of Yellow Pen Club,[1] play an essential role as well.

At times I am reminded of how writing, above all other things I do, is what *I* do. ~~If I'm not mistaken, I tend to be treated a lot better when participating in a project as a writer than in other roles.~~ But I have to admit that I am not the sole master of my writing, and I cannot insist on the pure and transparent authorship of what I produce. The environment, equipment, available fonts, ambience, references, online sources, things that happened during the day, what is playing in the background, directions I received, expectations of those involved: Writing is a collective dance of all these things.

6.

~~What time is it?~~ Everyone seems to have left the building already. The door is open. Quilts hang on the banister. I cannot believe I just slept the hours away. I felt drowsy the minute my usual dose of digital stimuli was removed. Had the state of being connected deprived me of sleep? Have I achieved inner peace? Have I become enlightened? What have I (not) done? I haven't received my phone yet, still slow with my senses. I have no idea what's going on in Seoul, if there's anyone looking for me, whether I've screwed something up without knowing, who twitted the dumbest thing today, which middle-aged man did something *naughty* this time, what Netflix has in store … ~~I don't know yet, and perhaps I don't really want to.~~

1. Yellow Pen Club is a collective of three writers who go by the pseudonyms Bbyabbya Kim, Looc, and Chongchong. Since 2016, Yellow Pen Club has written about topics related to the contemporary art scene, popular media, subculture, and literature—accessible at www.yellowpenclub.com. In pursuit of alternative modes of art writing and discussion, Yellow Pen Club organizes regular art writing workshops and reading groups.

Woochang Lee

Prison, Solitude, and the 'True Self'

1.

I enter the solitary confinement room. The door shuts behind me. Its length, from the entrance to the far wall with a window, is roughly 3 meters; its width 1.8 meters; and its height 2.5 meters. Excluding the parts occupied by the toilet, the entry aisle, and a very narrow wash-basin, the space given to the prisoner is about 3.4 square meters—just enough for an adult male to lie down. In the corner, there is a small drawer with four compartments to store simple belongings. An electric kettle and tea set rest on the windowsill. On a small table measuring the length of my forearm, writing materials and notebooks have been placed.

Apart from the short ring of a bell every hour, the only sound is a rainstorm. (It's the middle of the rainy season.) I'm left undisturbed until the following day, except for when a light dinner comes through a small slot at the bottom of the door. I fall asleep for a while, and when I wake up, the sun has already gone down. I turn on the light, and the window reflects the prisoner like a mirror. I turn it off, and darkness fills the space. My eyes, growing accustomed, can vaguely see the scenery outside the window: the grey sky and the dim hillside. After staring blankly for quite a while, I realize that I can't fall back asleep, so I come to think about what's left. A narrow space, a landscape that barely changes (except for some branches rocking in the wind), and myself with only memory, consciousness, and body—disconnected from society. These are all that are left.

Of course, the purpose of Happitory is not only to

provide a negative experience through the exclusion of many aspects of life. If we look closely at various practices proposed by the organization, we soon realize that this 'prison' also intends to have positive dimensions. Prisoners are trained to meditate, breathe, bow, and be Zen before entering their cells. They receive notebooks with prompts to consider how they might better organize their lives. It's important to note that these acts of governing and reflecting on body, mind, and memory are directed at a specific point—'I,' the self—as clearly shown by the language that permeates Happitory: the title of the program is "A Day to Meet *Myself*," and the notebook is labelled "Escaping the prison inside *me*" (emphases mine). In other words, Happitory tasks us to investigate and document ourselves in a space blocked from external, especially social demands. The goal is to find and restore the 'true self.'

Some would agree that such tasks are necessary for modern people, while others may criticize how imprisonment in a peaceful self-jail distracts us from seeing more essential issues. For me, there are other questions to ask: Why and how did we come to think that the 'true self' exists—and that we should seek it? Which moral ontology is premised on this belief? What kinds of technologies do we employ to become objects for questioning, exploring, and correcting? Since it is difficult to answer all of these questions comprehensively, this essay has a much smaller objective. First, I will look at self-inquiry and some traditions of what Michel Foucault calls the "care of the self." Then, I will consider how attempts to restore the 'true self,' such as

Happitory's program, can be a meaningful extension of those traditions.

2.

Let's start with philosophy. We usually think of philosophy as the subject of difficult books and works that reflect on the 'deep' truth of life. However, such an understanding only partly captures how it was practiced in the past. In the Classical period, according to Pierre Hadot, philosophy—above all else—referred to a specific way of life.[1] One strove to shape oneself into a complete being; philosophy was the collection of skills and knowledge necessary to achieve this goal.

In ancient Greece and Rome, it was believed that people could develop their capabilities through proper training, and that only those who learn to control themselves could rule their communities as excellent citizens. Based on the same logic, philosophers thought that training their bodies, minds, and souls in the 'right way' was required for philosophical life—though schools had different opinions about what this 'right way' entailed. Stoics and Platonists focused on the following point: the philosopher must, above all else, be a free being. (Here, being free meant establishing mastery over oneself.) The philosopher must also focus on the present moment, honing their concentration—through practices like meditation and memorization—in order to better comprehend themself and the world. If successful, they will eventually ascend to a mystical state, becoming one with universal principles.

We can observe characteristics from this philosophical tradition that continue into the early modern period. First and foremost, the human self is divided into parts. One part manages the other, training it to follow commands while minimizing the influence of negative internal and external factors. This task is not only important for taking care of the self: it can also boost, expand, and direct the self toward a higher realm. In that sense, a trained self can be a pathway for humans to enter a more genuine, worthy, even eternal world.

As Peter Brown shows, the fathers and monks of the early Christian era tried to refine and keep their bodies and souls in exemplary condition.[2] To do so, they drew on the rich intellectual resources of the aforementioned tradition. They were also deeply influenced by an influx of ascetics and penitents from the deserts of the Orient. Christians, in turn, added dimensions: for instance, they expanded the scope of self-control by inventing the construct of sexuality. Sexuality lurks within everyone and is a most powerful adversary, which can bring even the most virtuous person to their knees. Various methods for investigating and purifying the dark parts that lie within humans could be justified for the sake of countering them.

According to Foucault,[3] if Greco-Roman self-care demanded a person be their own master, the Christian model took a more social form, arguing that *all* human beings could and must approach God through faith and obedience. Despite this difference, both believed in the moral capacity of the self and the possibility of elevating it—and, above all, desired to connect with a transcendent realm. In fact, Christians widely cited writing by ancients like the Stoics and the 6th-century philosopher Boethius, who described meeting the female personification of philosophy during a period of imprisonment. Later in the 17th and 18th centuries, when Stoic writings were widely translated, it was easy to find authors who embraced the philosophy for portraying a life devout Christians should pursue.

3.

One of the traces left for future generations by Stoic philosophers like Marcus Aurelius and Seneca was the high status of solitude in philosophical life. In this tradition, solitude made it possible to separate oneself from the complicated matters of the mundane world, creating conditions to take a closer look at one's memories and life—and making it easier to correct mistakes. Consider the writing of Mary Chudleigh, a female intellectual of the late 17th century inspired by Stoic thinkers: loneliness, in her opinion, allows us to focus on self-discipline and the practice of faith. This belief continued to play an important role even in the Enlightenment, when the sociable nature of the human was emphasized more than ever. Jean-Jacques Rousseau's unfinished *Reveries of a Solitary Walker*, for one, contrasts the unjust and chaotic world with tranquil solitude.

So-called 'Romantic' literature made a significant

contribution to inscribing the image of the lonely self in western culture. What I want to emphasize here is not the loneliness of the self but the unique characteristics of the object with which it comes into contact. One ideal of 18th-century European culture was having a 'social life' with other members of 'civilized' society. It is thus unsurprising that periodicals like *The Spectator* and epistolary novels by Samuel Richardson became popular. However, we should remember that 18th-century Europeans were also deeply interested in 'uncivilized' worlds: the 'savage' New World; the world of their 'barbarian' and 'gothic' past; and the 'natural' world with few signs of human life. Reports by people who traveled outside Europe were read broadly, and history books about countries and ethnicities of the past frequently published. Popular demand fed various literary genres, including Gothic fiction and Romanticism, which were often marked by the encounter between the lonely self and the 'other' world.

Take the 1807 lyric "The Solitary Reaper," written by William Wordsworth. A narrator traveling in the Scottish Highlands encounters a woman singing and harvesting alone in a field. In the late 18th century, the region was a popular tourist destination for being 'not yet civilized.' Instead of trying to understand what her song means, the traveler, who might not have known the language of the Highlands, makes various associations while listening. Among them are exotic places (to the English reader) such as "Arabian Sands" and "the farthest Hebrides." Some lines link the past to the present to an open-ended temporality: "battles long ago," "Familiar matter of today," "Some natural sorrow, loss, or pain, / That has been, and may be again." The narrator, after listening to a song that seems to go on endlessly, continues up a hill, remarking: "The music in my heart I bore, / Long after it was heard no more."

In Wordsworth's poem, a traveler encounters a force that is almost transcendent—or at least, beyond what he has known in daily life in the 'civilized' world. His experience shares something with the aforementioned philosophical and Christian beliefs in the advance of the self and the unity of transcendent existence. If, in those traditions, such states are the result of constant spiritual training and self-discipline, in Romantic texts, the loneliness of the self and its encounters with other worlds are only conditions that make them possible.

4.

Another system of self-discipline we must address is the prison. Among the most well-known models is Jeremy Bentham's panopticon, conceived in the late 18th century. This circular prison, where the guard can see the prisoner but not the other way around, is often understood as a symbol of the modern nightmare that completely neutralizes the incarcerated. However, Bentham's intention was not to subjugate the prisoner but to build a 'school,' the surveillance system being just one of the means to 'educate' inmates. The goal was to reform prisoners into virtuous members of society, with appropriate social skills and diligence to fully participate in the workforce and community life. Bentham's endeavor was in keeping with moral philosophy and historical theory of the age, which sought to grasp the principles of how humans and society operate. It reflected the belief that, by employing these principles in the service of reformation, the panopticon could bring about the best outcomes consistent with justice and virtue.

Bentham's plan can be seen as a highly developed derivative of the self-discipline tradition, in that it promotes self-improvement through a thorough analysis of the human subject and the establishment of an appropriate 'corrective' environment. The subject I want to discuss runs counter to the panopticon and can be found particularly in modern Korean history. From the 1960s to the early 1990s, Korean society coexisted with a military dictatorship and the intensive and persistent movement against it. The dictatorship didn't tolerate those who threatened its control, so it was routine for politicians and intellectuals to be tortured, imprisoned, and confined. Of particular interest are cases in which imprisoned dissidents accepted prison life not only as a passive experience of the deprivation of liberty but an active opportunity to develop themselves. Their perceptions and practices, shared with fellow inmates and peers, were also conveyed to readers nationwide through the publication of prison letters.

Within this genre in Korea, the most widely known work is Kim Dae-jung's *Prison Writings*. The first edition, published in 1984, contained letters to family and colleagues that Kim wrote while imprisoned by the regime from 1980 to 1982. The popularity of the book owes, in part, to the author's later biography: After suffering numerous crises and hardships as a politician who criticized the regime, Kim was elected president and served from 1998 to 2003. Kim's extensive reading list and intellectual reflections left a deep impression on many readers. The fact that he was able to study while imprisoned, in a manner comparable to college, led later political prisoners to believe in the possibility of intellectual growth behind bars. It's interesting to note that Kim devotes a large part of *Prison Writings* to the Christian perspective. Confession of faith is one of the most frequently repeated themes; Kim writes that faith in the Absolute and dialogue with Him were the driving forces for enduring solitary life. The belief that he must accept his suffering as part of God's mission—and that he must strive to realize the will of God—show that, to him, the reign of the self and unity with a transcendent being are linked.

The ethical aspect of the Korean democratization movement is better illustrated in prison writing by those who clearly accepted the tenets of national populism (*Minjung-ism*). Shin Young-bok, who was sentenced to life imprisonment in 1968 for the 'Tonghyukdang case' and ended up serving twenty years, published *Reflections from Prison* in 1988. The work is celebrated for its elegant essay style. Kim wrote his letters in solitary confinement as a believer, head of household, and political leader; in contrast, Shin, imprisoned in his twenties as a university lecturer, lived with other inmates, assuming the identity of 'populist intellectual' in their midst. Instead of seeing such people as lowly members of society, Korean populism viewed them as subjects who suffered and were persecuted yet possessed unique strength and virtue vital for the nation's development and liberation. Shin thus felt that it was crucial to do more than study them, recognize their virtues, and foster their political awakening: he must unite in solidarity with them. In *Reflections from Prison*, Shin repeatedly mentions what he was not teaching but *learning* from the inmates right next to him—and how vain and lacking was the knowledge imparted by the upper-class world of college. Through this prison education, he refined and enlightened himself. At the same time, democratic activists like Shin were able to transform prison into a place for the populist care of the self.

Moon Ik-hwan devoted himself to democratization and the reunification of North and South Korea. In 1976, he was imprisoned for his dissident activities and spent more than ten years behind bars. Moon's prison writing is an interesting case of the intersection of Christian thought, national populism, and the care-of-the-self tradition. He was a Presbyterian pastor (like his father) who believed the history of the human world unfolded according to the will of God. And he did not see any problem in the coexistence of Christianity and nationalism, as he thought the reunification of the nation and the liberation of the people would come about by that will. Imprisonment was an invaluable experience for Moon, in that he learned to harmonize his faith with the nationalist and democratic movements. He also developed a yoga practice, which was as significant and ongoing as Kim Dae-jung's confession of Christianity. Through it, Moon came to realize that the matter of the self—from the unity of the body and the mind, to the macroscopic scale of national history—were not separate from one another. Yoga was the art of approaching dimensions small and grand through self-discipline.

In the 1990s, with the end of military dictatorship and the establishment of a democratic system, it was inevitable that populism, as an anti-regime movement, would gradually lose its power. Today, there are still some people who talk about the necessity of populist practice, but it is seldom discussed seriously in the Korean public sphere. Nevertheless, it is worth remembering that populism was not a mere political ideology but contained an ethical dimension that could be quasi-religious: people on the lowest rung of society were given the position of the highest, and intellectuals could approach them through moral and spiritual training. The self-disciplinary aspect of populism was powerful enough to turn even a long prison life into a course of spiritual practice. That said, the prison as 'school' gradually lost its spiritual connotation, ending when the former resistance entered the political mainstream.

5.

At the heart of Happitory's confinement program lies the traditional model of self-governance—especially the practice of exploring and managing oneself. Its prescribed activities (such as meditation, breathing, and the Buddhist ritual of 108 bows) are not just physical manipulations but exercises that control the mind via the body, leading one to a state of tranquility. Once the self has achieved this state, where should it be guided? Some insight can be found in the notebooks that Happitory provides for self-reflection. Participants are asked to graph experiences of happiness and unhappiness in their lives; draw their happiest and unhappiest moments; record important life events chronologically; and so on. Their lives are reorganized and simplified based on happiness and unhappiness. For instance, the prompt to draw "what you want to do most if you live for just one more year" sounds like a command to focus only on the pursuit of happiness by excluding all but the most important and most wanted things. A different prompt requests an "intermediate trial" of participants' lives from the standpoint of prosecutors, lawyers, and judges, asking "what is your inner prison that hinders your happiness?" It advises finding the factors that impede the realization of happiness, then removing them. Finally, a prompt to write a letter to yourself in your eighties compels participants to think about their future happiness. In short, the request to condense the past, remove unnecessary obstacles, and think about how to get closer to a happy state: this is the essence of the program. The 'true self' refers to a *purified* self that is only directed toward happiness. Prison is the *dispositif* for producing happiness at Happitory—quite literally, a 'happiness factory.'

Happitory's program differs from the traditions of self-discipline that we have surveyed thus far. Those traditions go beyond the mere shaping of the self in the name of greater philosophical, spiritual, or other goals. To borrow a line from George Eliot's *Middlemarch*, they endeavor that one not just live a better life but pursue "life beyond self."[4] The philosophical training at Happitory does not share this degree of ambition. Its solitary experience treats the self not as a means or medium but an end-in-itself. Ruling yourself is your happiness.

I have no intention of evaluating whether this form of self-discipline is problematic or harmful. In the present age—especially in Korean society, where no religion (not even Christianity) has succeeded in becoming hegemonic—the pursuit of transcendence is generally dismissed as a bizarre and irrational act. Perhaps for this reason, manifestations of self-discipline in contemporary culture often come stripped of mythical associations (for example, ridiculous 'personal growth' shows like Netflix's *Too Hot to Handle*), leaving little more than inflated self-care. I am left to wonder: Can such an overgrown ego gain the form and purpose to satisfy our aspiration for self-advancement, or will we create or rediscover a transcendent world only after this period ends? As a person who leans one arm against a thing called 'history,' I likely won't be surprised by either outcome.

1. See Pierre Hadot's *Philosophy as a Way of Life: Spiritual Exercises from Socrates to Foucault*, trans. Michael Chase (Oxford: Blackwell, 1995) and *What Is Ancient Philosophy?*, trans. Michael Chase (Cambridge, MA: Harvard University Press, 2002).

2. Peter Brown, *The Body and Society: Men, Women, and Sexual Renunciation in Early Christianity*, 2nd ed. (New York: Columbia University Press, 2008).

3. See Michel Foucault, *Histoire de la sexualité. IV: Les aveux de la chair*, ed. Frédéric Gros (Paris: Gallimard, 2018).

4. George Eliot, *Middlemarch* (1871; New York: W. W. Norton & Company, 2000), 3.

Sunjin Kim

A Worldview from Solitary Confinement

Aristotle Onassis visited the city of Daejeon with Nintendo's COO for a potential buyout of a kimchi fermentation lab. He fell in love with a retired women's volleyball player who was working at the lab and eloped to Fukuoka on an LNG carrier. A Mongolian archer presided over the wedding, which was held in a ryokan.

This is my mnemonic device, containing all the keywords that demand my attention. My original plan for solitary confinement was to put this device to work, but not long after the cell door locked, I fell asleep. The cell was dead quiet, and its floor was heated to a warm temperature. The scenery outside the window was breathtakingly beautiful. Immersed in the stillness of it all, my brain activity started slowing down. Rapid eye movement followed. Where one can feel no change, one can't perceive the flow of time. That's how I glided into sleep mode.

Inside the cell, there's no smartphone, no books. Just a pen and a notepad. I know of some great men in the history of humankind who became extremely smart during the time spent in prison. But I suspect they had access to books. And I do not. What am I supposed to write on this generic-looking notepad? My stream of thought? I need access to some type of information: an input that can elevate my output, sharpening the edge of my consciousness.

In a recent YouTube video, Charlie Munger bragged about his 'inversion thinking.'[1] I could apply that here. What if no-input isn't no-input? What if I have an input and am just not aware of it yet? What if the perceived poverty is in reality an abundance?

I began assessing my possessions: the mnemonic device I prepared from home, a lifetime's worth of memories, two eyes, two working legs, the giant untapped well of my subconscious, a Shinhan Bank credit card in my pocket, and some coins.

Some coins.

An idea flashed into my mind. I know what I will do. I can toss these coins and consult the old Asian oracle on the most difficult mysteries of our time. Luckily, I am well-acquainted with the method of the *I Ching* thanks to months of concentrated practice in 2019, when I was a budding value investor seeking accurate ways to narrow down my stock picks. More than anything, the poetic headline excites me: "summoning the ancient wisdom of the *Book of Changes* from inside a cell where one can't sense any change." Now I can say with certainty that Munger's inversion trick works.

The teachers of the *I Ching* instruct that one must remain respectful throughout the course of the consultation. I took my time carefully choosing my first inquiry. The big issues that occupy my Google News feed these days include the rise of nationalism and authoritarianism, the pandemic, and hegemonic struggles. Globalism as we know it seems headed for a change, so I think it deserves to be my first question: if globalism weakens and free trade diminishes, will Korea experience a food crisis?

> [Hexagram 7] The army retreats to the camp and no blame. Resistance brings misfortune.[2]

I have no idea why the *I Ching* is giving me a war reference. I asked about the future of free trade. During the coin toss, I pictured a fleet of cargo ships crossing the Pacific Ocean—and an avocado orchard in Peru. Carl Jung, who was a fervent student of this ancient technique, once stated (if I'm remembering correctly) that psyche and matter are not separated, and that psychic events and events happening in the outside world may influence each other. Maybe I had wanted to ask about war, but my psyche got shy and asked about the food crisis instead. Or maybe my subconscious fear of war interfered with the process.

Richard Wilhelm, a sinologist and *I Ching* expert of the early 20th century, explains the meaning of this hexagram as follows: "In the face of a superior opponent, an orderly retreat will save the army from defeat and disintegration."[3] Perhaps the *I Ching* is saying that countries should consider what they've got to lose before playing chicken. But one doesn't need to consult an oracle to know that recklessness is bad for business.

I feel the need to rephrase my initial question. I ask again: will we run into a food crisis within the next fifteen years?

> [Hexagram 51] The thunder terrifies a hundred miles and one does not lose the sacrificial spoon and chalice.

This is pretty literal. I thought the oracles were supposed to be subtle. No further questions on the topic.

My next question is about electric cars. I have been startled many times by electric vehicles silently sneaking up on me in the street. Lately, governments and manufacturers talk a lot about the discontinuation of gasoline cars by the 2030s. I'd like to know what's going on.

> [Hexagram 12] Inferior folks flock to the authority figure. Good fortune for the inferior. A setback serves to help the great man in the end.

This is very cryptic. What do palace politics have to do with the future of the car industry? Who's the "authority figure," who are the "inferior folks"? And who is this "great man"? My guess would be that Tesla is the "authority figure." A myriad of auto parts companies, battery manufacturers, bitcoin fanatics, long and short traders, and journalists flock to Elon Musk's Twitter feed. I presume "the great man" represents the traditional automakers. They have it all: mass-production capabilities, production speed, supply chains, and sales networks. Tesla occupies most of the "inferior folks'" attention, which can be viewed as a setback for the traditional automakers, but the *I Ching* suggests the situation may change with time. In the end, they may reclaim their lost authority through the electric vehicle market.

So electric vehicles are the future of cars? Does this mean that fathers working on family cars over the weekend won't smell like gas and engine oil anymore?

> [Hexagram 53] The wild goose gradually draws near the shore.

Wild geese are migratory birds. They come and go. You see them one season, and they're gone the next. Why do wild geese draw near the shore? To have the last feast before departing for a new summer house. This oracle is suggesting that gasoline cars will go. And fathers may not reek of gas and engine oil in the future.

Would this change the demand for crude oil? What will happen to the oil-rich Middle Eastern countries?

> [Hexagram 55] The curtain cast over the abundance. Dark. The North Star is visible at high noon. One meets a like-minded leader and things will improve.

This oracle's level of symbolism is not very profound. The curtain is drawn over oil-rich nations, and the future looks dark. On the bright side, those in trouble may have a chance for a turnaround once they find the right partnership. But to cross over to the bright side, one must walk the dark side first. I would say that the *I Ching* is pessimistic in the short-term but optimistic in the long-term.

Now I'll change the subject and ask about the art world. First and foremost, I hear the word NFT a lot. That's the biggest development since I began distancing myself from the art world after the outbreak of Covid-19. I've done some homework. NFT is short for non-fungible token. Non-fungible means the token is not interchangeable. Though NFTs were designed using the same blockchain-based technology as cryptocurrencies, they're not a cryptocurrency because they're not a currency. For a currency to function as such, it needs to have units that one can add, subtract, merge, and divide. NFTs don't have units because their tokens are not uniform.

An artwork published via NFT technology is given a unique digital marker certifying the work's authenticity, without the need to involve a central art-world authority. Does this make NFTs good for art?

> [Hexagram 23] The leg of the bed is split. Those standing are destroyed. Misfortune.

Any broken leg is bad news, even the leg of a bed. A bed is a support for a human body, and the bed's leg is a support for the bed. This oracle is implying that the NFT is a leg-breaker: a destroyer of fundamentals. The fundamental of an NFT would be the artwork underlying and authenticated by the token. In short, NFTs will destroy art.

Public response to the NFT seems divided: for some, it offers novel opportunities to capitalize on art, while for others, it threatens the established order of things. Will this mania die down? If so, how?

> [Hexagram 4] To enlighten the young and foolish. It furthers one to apply discipline. To proceed without fetters makes things worse.

The *I Ching* and I are on the same page here. Change always stirs up fear of the unknown. The question is who's going to pick up the spanking bamboo. The sellers of NFT art? Its buyers? The ousted middleman?

The whole fuss seems to come from the NFT's power to authenticate an artwork's uniqueness without the mediation of art institutions. Honestly, I don't understand why uniqueness even matters at this time in history. Uniqueness is not synonymous with value. Does the NFT's non-fungibility really add anything new?

> [Hexagram 9] An image of incremental accumulation. Favorable. Clouds thicken from the West. No sign of rain yet.

I am silently blown away by the fact that the *I Ching* just produced an oracle in accord with Marcel Duchamp's concept of *infrathin*. Within a cloud, water droplets begin to grow. As the cloud gets denser, they become heavier and heavier, building to a critical moment when the very first droplet, now too heavy to stay suspended, starts to fall—an *infrathin* moment.

The oracle's Duchampian nuance reminds me of Jorge Luis Borges's short story "Pierre Menard, Author of the *Quixote*." Menard wished to "compose *the* Quixote," putting tremendous effort into the endeavor.[4] The resulting work is identical to the original Cervantes, word for word—different only in an imperceptible manner.

As the *I Ching* points out, the non-fungible side of

NFT art feels somewhat retro. It's an age-old concept accidentally revived through new cryptotechnology. I'm not suggesting we shouldn't use the token. I'm just saying I'm going to ignore it for a little longer.

Right after finishing this part of the consultation, I fell asleep again. Asking the *I Ching* eight questions in a row involved forty-eight consecutive coin tosses. The act of coin tossing is like exploring the terrain of one's subconscious—and looking into my subconscious was massively exhausting. The nap was unavoidable. Also, the cell was awfully quiet, and the floor was warm.

I woke up at the sound of a prison guard yelling in the corridor. It was the next morning. The guard was yelling at the inmates. An orderly exit was the message he was trying to convey. It was time to leave solitary confinement. I was dismayed at the fact that my consultation was cut short by my untimely sleep. I hadn't gotten to half the questions I wanted to ask.

The yelling of the guard was getting louder by the second. The pressure was growing. I remember thinking to myself that I must finish strong—this would be my way of paying respect to the 5,000-year-old book of wisdom—even though I knew there was absolutely no way that I could get through the rest of my questions. It was time for acceptance and damage control.

As I've mentioned, it is advised that a practitioner of the *I Ching* remain respectful until the very end of a consultation (bad mojo if this rule isn't followed) so I managed to toss the coins six more times before the guard flung open the door, saw me playing with the coins, and started harassing me. My final question to the *Book of Changes*: do you have any advice for today's artists?

> [Hexagram 10] A one-eyed man is able to see. A lame man is able to tread. He treads on the tail of the tiger. The tiger bites the man. Misfortune. Thus does a warrior act on behalf of his great king.

What is a one-eyed man most desperate to do? To see clearly with his one eye. What is a lame man most desperate to do? To walk straight despite his lameness. When desperate men try too hard to prove their capabilities, they make important people angry, defeating the purpose of their efforts. An artistic warrior's goal must be to serve something larger than themself—and never to exhibit their capabilities just for the sake of it.

1. “Charlie Munger: The mental models I used to become successful in life,” YouTube video, 29:07, January 8, 2021, https://www.youtube.com/watch?v=ZuHHmVX8a00.

2. All hexagrams in this text were translated by the author from Tae-Yeon Hwang’s *The Positive I Ching* (Seoul: Chunggye, 2008).

3. Richard Wilhelm, “I Ching,” http://www2.unipr.it/~deyoung/I_Ching_Wilhelm_Translation.html.

4. Jorge Luis Borges, “Pierre Menard: Author of the *Quixote*,” in *Collected Fictions*, trans. Andrew Hurley (1939; New York: Penguin Books, 1999).

Jaeyeon Chung

1.

When I was in middle school, my whole class had to participate in a choir contest, because the homeroom teacher taught music.
We sang a song called *Nostalgia* based on Jeong Ji-yong's poem of the same name.
If there were any mistakes, they quickly became noticeable, so I tried hard to memorize the lyrics.
I could even imagine the situations they described.

How many times have I sung that song, since coming to this facility?
I dare to write the lyrics down, trusting my memory:

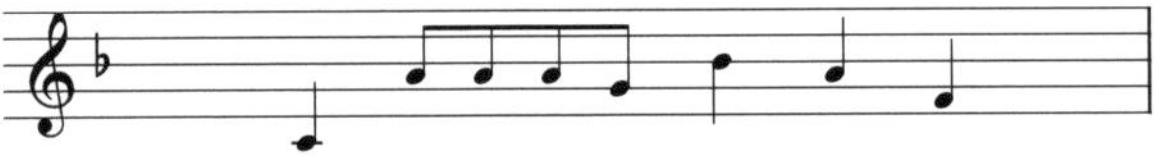

To the east end of the vast field

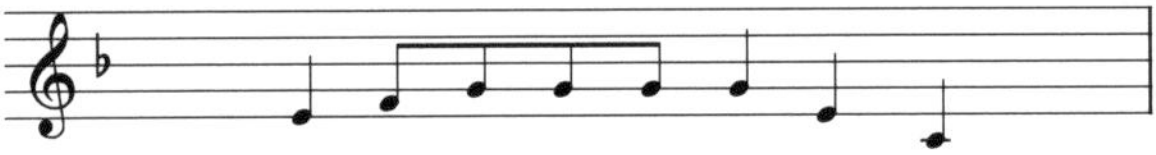

Where old legends were told

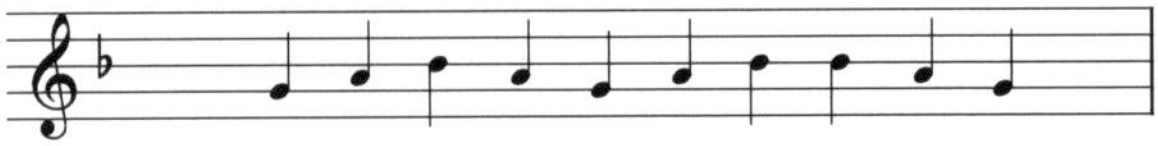

A streamlet was meandering.

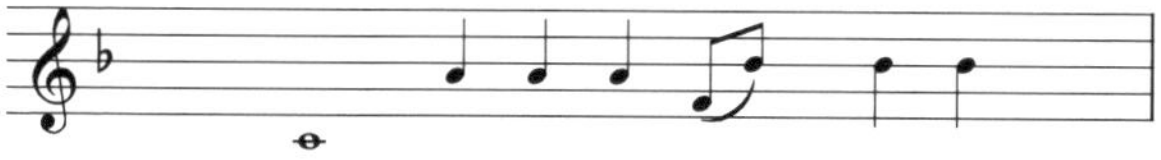

And spotted oxen

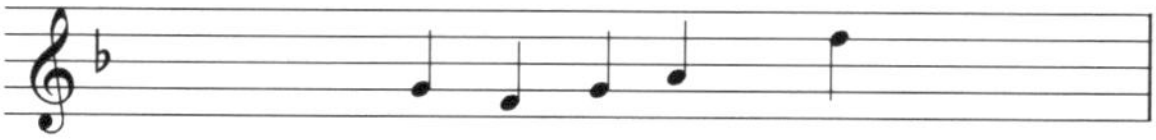

Were lowing peaceably

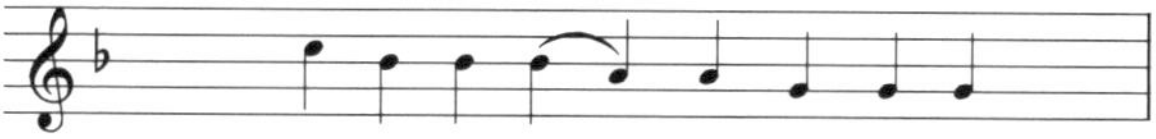

Their lazy golden calls

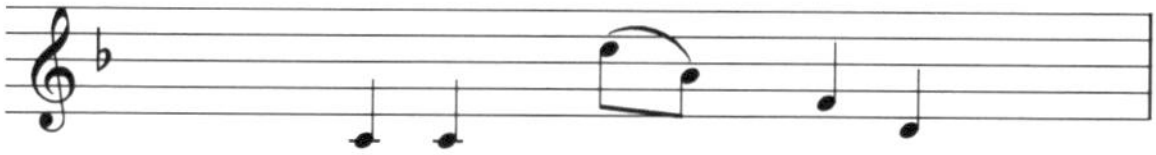

Such a place,

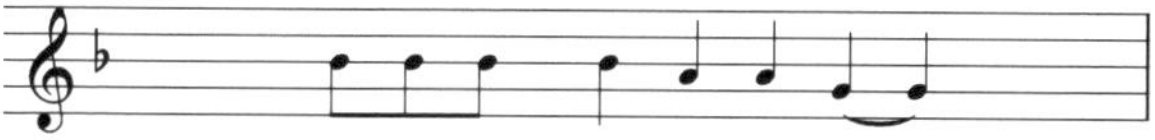

Will ever be forgotten, even in a dream

As expected, the first measure sticks in my throat.
I vividly remember the melody; however, the lyrics are blurry.

The first and second verses are all mixed up and deviate from the pitch.
The refrain is awkward.
If I were home, I could correct this right away with a single internet search …
(I turned over my smartphone just before entering this room.)

I struggle again and again to piece the lyrics together.
I combine the words that have come up so far and sing them in my mind.
I would like to sing them loudly if I could.
But it is obvious that I will regret it tomorrow, when I encounter the person staying in the next room.
In the end, I sing the song in a low whisper (preserving my dignity).
Oh, it seems the words and syllables that weren't in place become clearer.
It feels like the narrative, and the combination of words that have been wandering about, fit little by little:

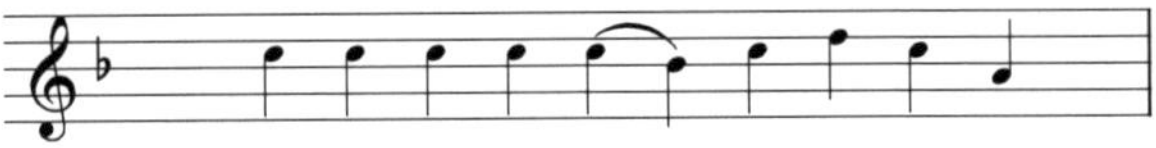

When ashes in the clay brazier became cool

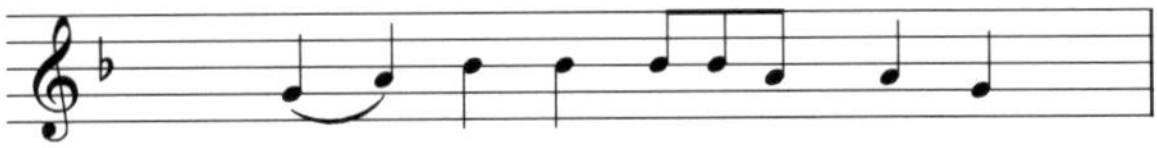

Sounds of night winds ran across

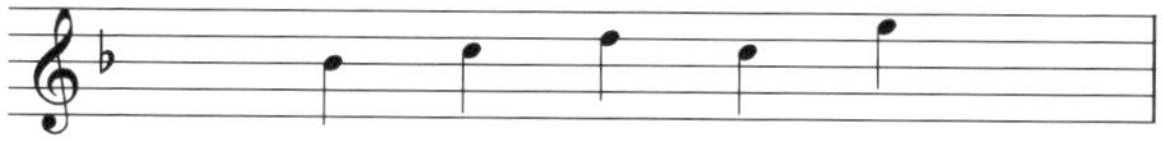

From the empty fields

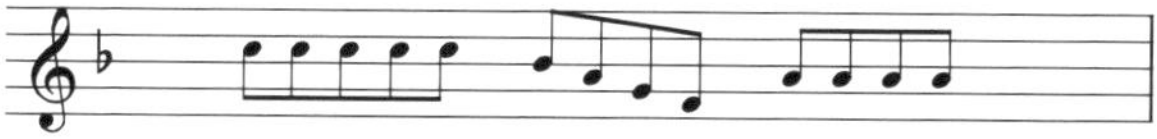

Autumn crows flying, cawing sadly

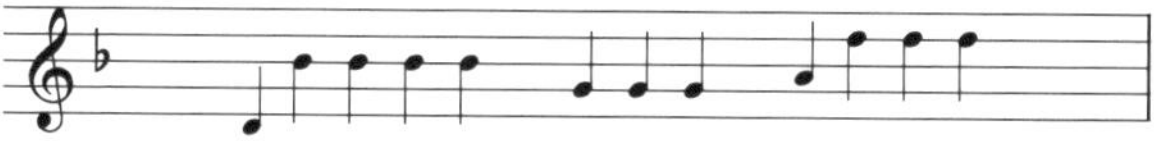

....

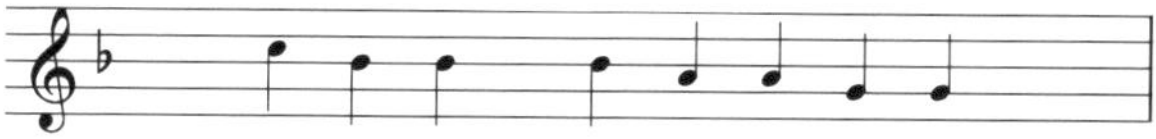

....

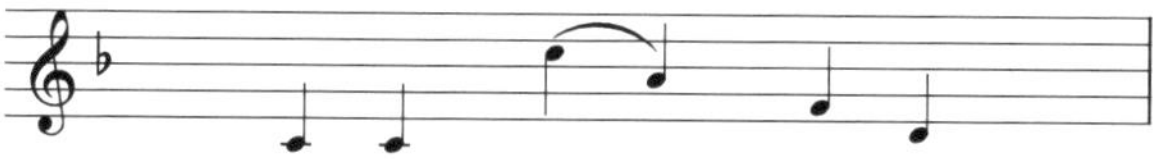

Such a place,

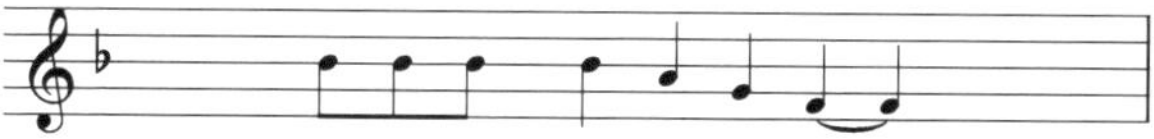

Will ever be forgotten in a dream?

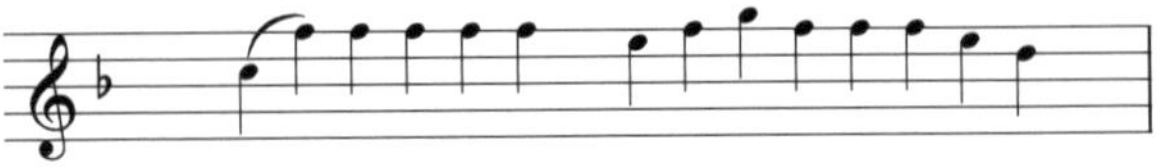

Dancing like night waves in the legendary sea,

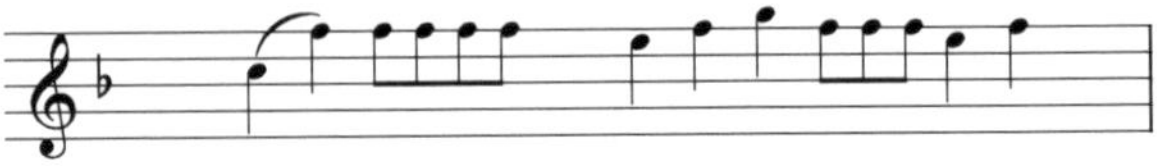

My baby sister, whose dark brown hair blown away,

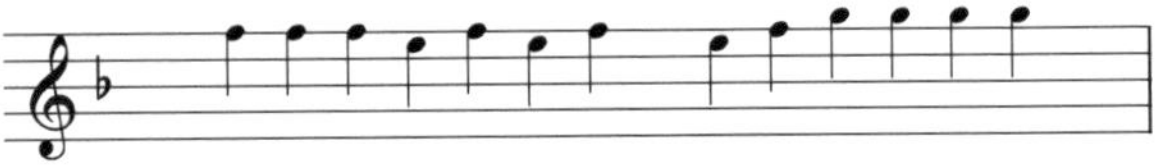

And my plain-looking and not-so-pretty

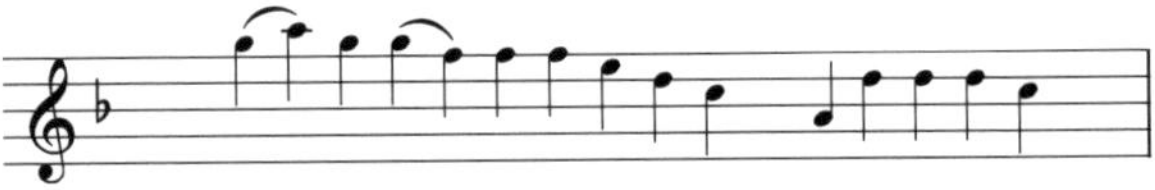

Wife always barefoot ....

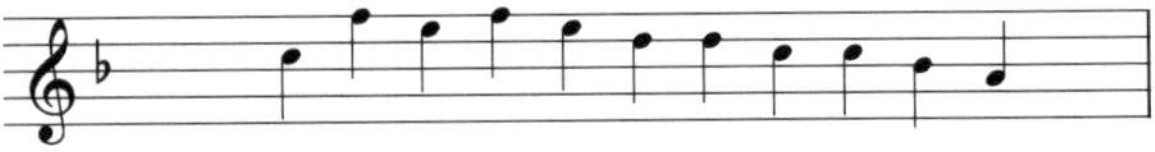

Were gleaning grains

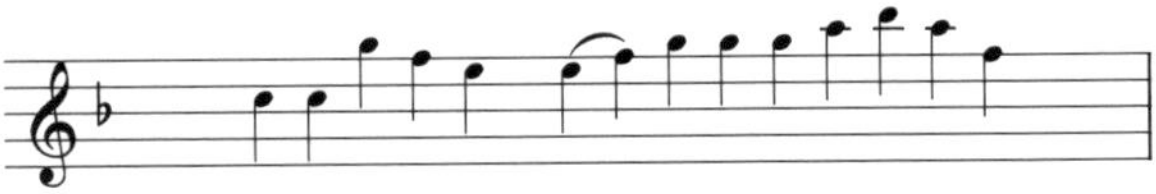

Such a place, will ever be forgotten even in a dream?

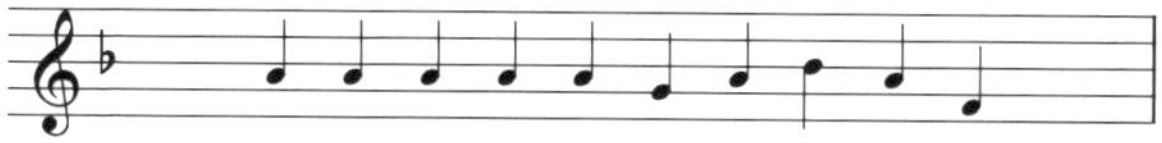

In the sky, stars far apart

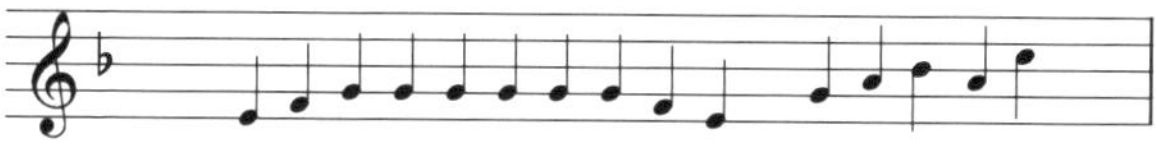

Moving toward unknown sandcastles, a horse runs

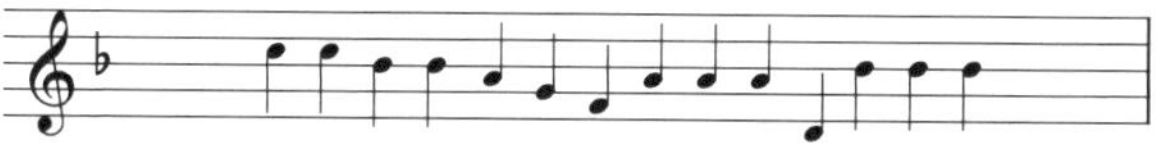

And aged father dozing off and on

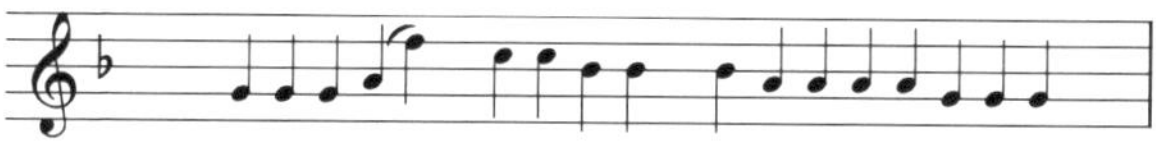

Tried to raise his straw pillow up and straight

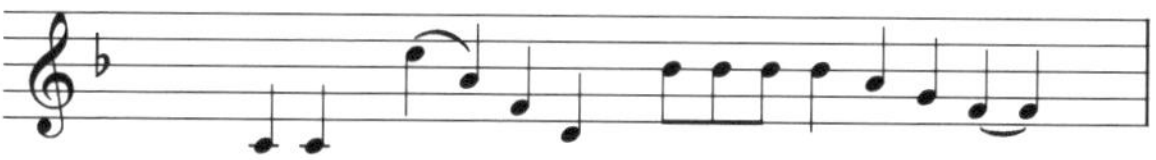

Such a place, will ever be forgotten even in a dream?

2.

It suddenly became dark outside the window.
I don't remember the lyrics in their entirety yet, but it's too hard to recall the rest of them.
I hurry to conclude that the process itself was meaningful enough.

What do I do now?

In fact, there's no goal to achieve during my time here. Rather than expect a solitary confinement experience, I thought this would be an opportunity to practice the "noble meditation of silence" that my husband follows. He's in another room at this facility; I want to make a memory with him while we're here.

Ever since my husband began to meditate, he goes to a meditation center each summer.
It appears that he becomes a completely different person after his stay.
His outlook turns positive, and his self-control grows.
His body gets lighter by suppressing the appetite that he usually can't resist.
As a result, it seems that his satisfaction with life increases, and he can enjoy some peace of mind.
However, this state has an expiration date.
If he feels like his body and mind are distracted, he starts meditating again.
Then he recovers the fullness.

For my husband, the purpose of meditation is to not think.
But is it really possible to exist without thinking?
I was most curious about that.
So I had some expectation that this room would enable me to experience an unthinking state.

But now that I'm here, I keep trying to do stuff whenever I can.
I continue to think about something.
I stare out the window constantly.

I hear a sound from outside.
It's a sign that it would rain soon.
I can hear raindrops flowing down the wires.
I can see a heron sitting on a branch and picking its feathers.
I can see the fog passing across the mountain and sky.
I can hear the footsteps of an officer quietly carrying a meal.
A grandfather clock awakens the stillness.

Oh, after experiencing all of this, will I remember the rest of the lyrics clearly?
By the way, where was Jeong Ji-yong's hometown?
I start to think again. It is so hard to not do anything.

Perhaps the creative process should begin from the premise that nobody is obliged to disclose what results, and it's useless to try to do so.

Russell Mason

Rain falls steadily outside, just as it has for the whole summer. I am locked inside a small room, though I am anything but concerned. For some time, I alternate between sitting and lying completely still. I feel the calm and silence of the space, both inside and outside my body, until the distinction between inside and outside no longer exists. I stare at the thicket of trees in front of me through half-open eyes. I focus on the emptiness of the scene and wait. When I hit the sweet spot, clear light floods in.

I remain motionless and totally at ease as everything I see fades from view; the image of my body also fades and flickers like a reflection on water. Now that the mind has come to a stop, my background awareness is foregrounded—shining. My being begins to intuitively heal itself. In the absence of any mental activity, there is bare existence and pacific relief, until I grasp at a persistent thought that draws me out of this ocean of bliss. Something is troubling me: the writing I have been asked to do in return for my stay.

With words spinning through my mind, I resolve to start. *Fulfill the terms of the agreement first, discharge this mental noise, then relax and focus on meditation.* The table in the room is extremely low and awkward to use, and I must decide whether my knees or elbows will bear the discomfort. I imagine the ease with which my Korean wife—and no doubt all the other Koreans staying at the facility—will take to it. As there is no internet connection, I'm writing with pen and paper. It has been many years since I've done this, and a skill once so fluid, practiced so ardently as a student, is now somehow unnatural. My brain circuitry seems to have undergone reverse plasticity, as I can barely form the shapes of letters. Writing has taken on the narrative arc of my sexual history: an unrelenting flow reduced to intermittent dribble.

Knowing the dangers of procrastination, I begin without forethought:

"What meditating and writing on a blank piece of paper have in common is that in both cases, we are forced to confront the content of our minds. The words that come to me as I write upon this page, like the words that are present to the mind in meditation, can be nothing other than my thoughts at this very moment."

Not bad, I reflect, but these are not your ideas: you merely internalized them from social discourse. I press on regardless.

"But what about the grass, the verdant trees, and the pale canvas of sky that I see through the window? Surely those are not thoughts in my mind. Those are objects in a real world out there, real things that occupy specific locations in time and space outside my body. Those could never be thoughts in my mind. Or is this merely an uninvestigated assumption?

"In point of fact, there can never be such a thing as a mind-independent view of the world. The trees, the falling white light, and the lazy stones are sense perceptions or sense-mediated images in my mind. No human being has ever seen the world, nor could they. All of us have only ever seen the content of our own minds and, in shared confusion, spoken or written about a concept or set of concepts called 'the world.' Despite this being totally and utterly obvious, nobody seems to really stop and consider it. Most persist in believing that the world of their own perception is an indubitably real object of experience outside the body, though the existence of such a world has never been and can never be proven; it is just an assumption that makes subsequent discussion meaningfully possible. But let's stop for a moment and see what we can make of this assumption.

"If we consider our waking life, we seem to either *be a body* or *be 'in' a body,* and that body experiences a world outside itself. There seem to be two basic facts: the body and what is inside it, and the world or universe outside it. But have we already made a false step? Have we needlessly added a second fact? On the basis of our experience, is there any certain ground or proof that establishes, beyond any reasonable doubt, that I am merely a body or 'in' a body and not simultaneously the ever-present space outside it as well? Most of us, of course, have firsthand experience of thoughts, feelings, sensations, and emotions that we speak of as our *interior* lives. Does this reveal anything more substantial than a habit of speech and an attachment to a concept of interiority? Without concepts of interiority and exteriority, sensations and emotions are still experienced; there is simply an awareness of a more extended continuum of feeling that does not stop at the boundary skin of the body. We are deeply attached to metaphors of containerization, so used to mapping worlds with ins and outs through culturally specific semiologies, and living our lives accordingly—like unopened tins of soup. Because we like the ins and outs too much, oceanic consciousness has shrunk to the condensed space beneath our skin."

As I finish writing this sentence, I become aware that the act of analyzing my thoughts has reduced my awareness of existence, making me incapable of experiencing the mode of consciousness I wish to express.

"As the body and the space outside the body are ever-present facts of our waking life, how do we *know* that we are merely one and not both? How do you *know*, at the most fundamental level, that you are even either of these things? The body and the universe both appear as objects of perception to us or perhaps within us. Can an entity appear as an object of perception to itself? Could you be the act or the process of knowing —perception itself—and witness all the forms, objects, and experiences that dissolve within the frame of time? If you are truly honest with yourself, you will admit that you *don't know*. And it is when you reach the point of admitting that you don't know, that you can never know, when you despair of ever knowing, when you surrender every effort to know, when you give up all the micro-dramas of the fake self you are so deeply attached to and in love with, that you are ready to know something more. Until this point, you are superimposing your idea of the world onto the world and living out that fantasy. Every effort you make is an investment in keeping the illusion going. You are dreaming that you are a separate self who understands the world.

"What are the root causes of this prison that most of us inhabit? It arises partly from a belief in separate objects. By focusing our attention on a specific 'interior' or 'exterior' object—a thought, sensation, pain, tree, or even a word—we immediately see that object as being separate from the rest of the universe which actually gives it context and meaning. This is not a trivial matter, because our basic mode of attention has us living in a near-continuous state of diversion toward such objects. It is the desire for a specific object, goal, fantasy, love object, or even fantasy love object that keeps us inhabiting the world of separation. In this sense, the prison is constructed out of our desires; fears and projections; and attempts and struggles to understand the world. By existing in default modes of pleasure-seeking and knowledge-seeking, we mistakenly suppose that objects exist outside us, become fascinated by one such object, then believe that it has fulfilled our desire when the craving for it temporarily ceases. Although repeated experience should tell us that the object never satisfies our desire, we don't learn this simple lesson. In fact, each object we seek is a secondary desire masquerading as our true desire for quiescence, which can only be achieved by relinquishing the pursuit of objects. Every action we take is done in the hope that it will be the last action—the final action, the one that enables the fruitless search to come to completion. But we can only experience our true nature once we give up looking for it in all these false substitutes."

And there it is. I have almost settled the issues plaguing the western mind for centuries, and I have not been here two hours. I can come back to this later. I certainly earned a reward: spending some time submerged in the lake of pure awareness.

I lie completely still and focus all my attention on my body. However, the relief I expect to feel does not materialize. I cannot really relax. I continue to ruminate, reading the text of my mind.

Gazing at the darkening sky, a thought suddenly occurs: *I cannot get out of the room.* I am not exactly panicking, but it carries an electric charge. I open the window and smell the fresh air. *You have to be in this room for another fifteen hours.* I look at the volunteers who work at the center walking around outside. Even though I have no desire to join them in the rain, I hate them for their freedom.

I sit for awhile, lost on board this useless train of thought, then notice how slowly time is passing. When the clock outside strikes the hour, I long for an extra stroke, growing too weary and listless to write or meditate.

Unexpectedly, I am filled with a desire to scream out in rage, to rattle and bang on the door to the room. My thoughts are caught in a downward spiral. I get a brief glimpse of the anger, boredom, and futility that people in prison must so often feel, but it is enough to gain an unmistakable insight: *being deprived of freedom is a punishment in itself.*

I turn the light off. I want to sleep as soon as possible. I want the day to be over. But as I lie in darkness, I wonder how difficult it must be to sleep in an actual prison. The threats imagined by an overactive mind can be unpleasant even at the best of times; how much worse must these be when multiplied by the very real threats faced by the incarcerated? I wait for the onset of sleep, but because I am willing this waiting, I remain awake for some time. Restless thoughts stumble around, like amateur burglars, until stolen away by the night.

I sleep surprisingly well. When I wake in the morning, I feel much less agitated than I did the previous night. The sound of the alarm is actually quite pleasant, like one of those musical boxes that might be used to help get a baby to sleep. As the sound continues, I look for an alarm clock but cannot find one anywhere. The noise, by this point, has become extremely annoying. I search for a button or switch on the wall, on the table top. My mind is racing, as it often does first thing in the morning: *I'm going insane from this ridiculous music piped into the room without my consent.*

After a few minutes, the sound stops, and a recorded voice begins, announcing that it's time for the 108 protestations. This Buddhist practice, common in South Korea, was strongly recommended by our hosts at Happitory. As the voice instructs, I begin to bow in my awkward and clumsy way, but my mind is full of resentment and anger. I decide I cannot continue until I am able to form an appropriate bearing of gratitude. I adopt the seated meditation posture and try to focus on images of the spiritual teachers who have greatly enhanced my life. I give thanks for Gautama Buddha, Lao Tzu, Padmasambhāva, Tilopa, Adi Shankara, and Meister Eckhart, and as I do so, my body opens to a warm current of energy from its heart center. Each time I offer my gratitude to Tenzin Wangyal Rinpoche, S.N. Goenka, Sayagyi U Ba Khin, and Ledi Sayadaw, a wave of love fills up the empty vessel of my body and merges with the space outside. I remember the meditation teachers and fellow students on the retreats I did at Dhamma Korea before the center closed due to the coronavirus outbreak. I think of Samaneri Jayasara, an Australian nun who offers free recordings of the most inspired discourses from the world's spiritual traditions. Then I decide to give thanks for the people in my life: for my wife, for each member of my English and Korean families, for my friends and mentors.

Although I've read about the importance of gratitude practices, and even tried to do them with some success, I have mainly been playing the game that most of us play: remembering to always express gratitude in speech, keeping a tally of the kindnesses done to me, and reciprocating in turn. This is nothing but the outer shell of gratitude. I can see now that what has been missing is the actual feeling of gratitude. As I give heartfelt thanks for these teachings, and for the people who have helped me so much in my life, wave after wave of something unmistakable rises from the depths of my unconscious mind, manifesting as knowledge of the interconnectedness of all life—sweeping away the lingering anxieties that were upsetting me. It is at once overwhelming and becalming.

When the recording of the 108 protestations concludes, I sit with newfound calmness and am struck by the clarity of some basic insights. This process of writing forced me back into an analytical mode of thinking. Despite my best efforts, I fell into the prison of mental activity, where the experience of being a separate body is utterly real. In this state of mind, it is impossible to realize the unity of consciousness. You might as well ask a drunk person to become sober by simply imagining it.

As these thoughts arise, the time and space between them extends, and the sequential nature of reality again fades away. The last one I can recall—as I sit here at home, several hours later, finishing this writing on my laptop—is that I should preface my text with a statement to the effect that nothing I want to say here can actually be said in words. This is actually why I gave up the fantasy of being a writer some years ago. Staying at Happitory has been not only an opportunity to relive that former incarnation of myself, but a convenient excuse to attempt to say what, in all honesty, cannot be said—long after I resolved never again to attempt to say it. As the memories of the room, the trees, and the rain slip away, I can affirm that, yes, I am also grateful for this.

InYoung Yeo

Curving the orgasm in organism

The surface is flat

The flat ***hole***[1] begins to end. At a dot, it pixel-izes into a squircle. Seven above begin to protrude. Eventually, they come to look three-dimensional. One part rotates. Two holes rotate one another. Three parts rotate each other. Four dots rotate in pairs and swap to rotate others. Two pairs of twos and threes rotate each other. Six group together and rotate in threes. Seven parts rotate within themselves and with each other. The rotation begins again. The axis changes its course, its path, a millimeter with each new beginning.

I think I'm rotating based on some point. Where is this in time and space? A hole, a ***part***,[2] a whole? Across it measures the same from its vertical point to point as its horizontal point to point. The whole count of holes comes to *twelve* holes in parts: (1,1,0,0), (1,0,1,0), (1,0,0,1), (0,1,0,1), (0,0,1,1), (0,1,1,0). One part breaks. One zero stays its course. Two work together, falling into holes until they become a ***whole***,[3] a big flat hole.

The surface is flat. The surface rotates, curves, bends, and folds. It's three-dimensional and continues to flatten.

A superegg is born.

1 : one is full of boxes, one is full of curves.

0 : let's start from the end.

1 : from your end or mine?
0 : from our end.
1 : the end goal is convenience.
0 : that's the beginning.
1 : that's one part, what about the whole hole?
0 : there are six sides to a box, how many sides does a whole hole have?
1 : a hole has a 360-degree curve.
0 : let's carve that curve into a thin slice and make a box out of it.

0 : I see.
1 : flatten out the sliced curve.

1 : I see one side.
0 : I see ***two sides***.[4]
1 : I see three sides.
0 : I see four sides.
1 : I see five sides.

0 : I see 0 side. I see the curve.
1 : simply cut the six sides of the box, spread it open, and fit it into the 360-degree curve in the hole.
0 : sure, is anything inside?
1 : everything is inside and everything is outside.
0 : the surface is ***transparency***,[5] semi-transparency, semi-opaque, opaque. It's reflect-ing, mirror-ing, spiral-ing, differ-ing, connect-ing, block-ing, absorb-ing ... 'i.n.g.'-ing.
1 : how deep is it?
0 : it dips internally, externally, horizontally, vertically,

diagonally, and in all directions on the surface and in depth.

1 : where do we meet?
0 : I meet you.
1 : I meet you.
0 : We meet.
1 : I meet, you meet, we meet, they meet me.
0 : where?

1 : one is full of boxes, one is full of curves.

Carving the flat to curve into the H'O'LE

The curves and flats lie out the sight. On the *hole* of my pupils, the curves dash. I check to see if I missed a light. Nothing stands still, and time starts to run again. Without a *tap* and a *click* and a *swipe*, I'm not sure what that means, so I look elsewhere. I find the greens and a friend that I can share with. I sit flat on the surface, the face curves around 360 degrees not laterally, not vertically nor horizontally but rather curiously. I flow onto the pool of water. Somehow the blue turns heavy and flips me over to the other side. I float to the top and sit, the curve starts to stop, and the body flattens in relation to the motionless *hole*. I look inward, and the colorful fingernails bend to meet. Finding it difficult to reach each other, they make a detour around and around to and from one another. As the routes and shapes create a new ***pattern***,[6] the thumb starts to thump, thump, thump. One thump, and the vibration is felt. It feels like an error or a coincidence, but maybe I meant it with all intention and with a flat goal to make and meet the ***desire***.[7]

I can't seem to touch you, so I pick up my best friend and touch everything I can. It doesn't feel warm but it's easy, convenient, and sometimes spectacular. As the face moves, flows, and orbits around my face, I simply de-face and face another face. The face-ing and de-face-ing layers into a flat wide curve I walk over. My close-ness is beyond, yet I then bend and ask.

2 : the goal is convenience.
0 : I see tiny holes.
1 : tiny holes? where?

1 : in my boxes.

0 : text me the ***information***,[8] let me find a question.
1 : the goal is to piss in the holes, collect the red x's, highlight the boxes, you are the holes.

1 : the stockings over the boxes, are they x's?
0 : I think they're yellow.
1 : assuming they're yellow with a goal to piss in the holes, does that mean you love my tiny holes?
0 : yes and no.

1 : scenario <yes>
0 : the hole is a dot.
1 : look at it close enough, and it's a flat black dot.

0 : the hole multiplies and grows into a whole.
1 : I love it when you multiply.
0 : put your face in the hole, what do you feel?
1 : it's rotating.
0 : de-face your face in numbers that lead and follow zeros and ones.
2 : the goal is convenience.

0 : scenario <no>
1 : the hole is no-thing.
0 : two thumbs for the two holes.
1 : perfect.
2 : the goal is convenience.

1 : scenario <zero>
0 : the hole is whole is hole in parts is whole and hole again.
1 : zero marks the start and end.
0 : it is infinite.
2 : the goal is convenience.

2 : the goal is convenience.

The 'O'rgasm in 'O'rganism

Fear *in* sensation of dying *out* of breath *in* torture *out* of patience *in* self. It feels like death, a never-ending death. Can you imagine? A never-ending death? Out of breath has never felt so alive.

Heat falls into place of *lust* and *pleasure* for content. Hot heated desire, seeing in all parts, as parts don't belong to a whole but to a hole. Weary and ***alienated***[9] from the walls, the windows, and the light, 'I fall asleep.' Real, more real than fake, more false than real. Not a single touch and a whole hole sensation, beyond and *around* it all. An 'Oh,' maybe the letter 'O' and the number '0' go *around* and *around*. Round and round. They go round and round in 360-degree dimension and return to 'nothing' where everything begins and ends and becomes 'whole' again with parts and holes.

0 : I'm ***loop***[10]-ing.
1 : I'm erecting. I'm penetrating. I'm colonizing.
The loop is mine. I win.
0 : I'm spiraling. I'm sharing. I'm emptying.
1 : I don't understand. It doesn't make sense.
0 : you're not the one and only signifier.
1 : I'm the answer.
0 : I'm full of questions. What's the next question?
Part, hole to whole, in the numbers that lead and follow ***zeros and ones***.[11]
1 : I see a windowless mirror, it reflects its power onto others filled with wonderful things.
0 : the mirror in me flows sticky yet soft, empty and translucent yet full, it reflects, reciprocates, cycles.
1 : what do I get?
0 : it's a loop, no one gets it and everyone gets something, it spirals.
1 : it loops so it starts with a new loop. I'd like an 'o,' a '0.'

0 : in the new loop is a spiral without an 'o' but multiplications of zeros and ones.

0 : it's an open spiral.
1 : I'd like an 'o.'
0 : I'd like an 'O.'
1 : I'd like a '0.'
0 : I'd like a hole.
1 : close the room.
0 : open the room.
1 : I'm loop-ing.

Spiraling in simulation [12]

The Script

0 : what's ***real***? [13]
1 : in *threes*,

1 : subject, mediator, object,
0 : ***whole***,[14] part, hole,
1 : observer, interpreter, receiver
0 : I'm *fascinated*.
1 : a face curves,
0 : it flattens,
1 : it's one face,
0 : it's zero and many faces, layers carved out into one face,
1 : it's one answer,

0 : it’s zero and many questions, answers carved out
into one answer,
1 : I’m confused,
0 : *I’m curious,*

0 : spiral back, what’s *real*?
1 : imagine ***hyperreality***,[15]
0 : zeros and ones,
1 : sur-faces,
0 : it *differs* to unite,
1 : ***organizing***[16] as the faces surface in differences,
0 : the flat curves as it diffracts,
1 : close the room,
0 : it flattens,
1 : open the room,
0 : it curves,
1 : ones and zeros,
0 : spiral back, what’s *real*?
1 : the capital ‘O’ in HOLE, WHOLE, ORGASM,
and ***ORGANISM***,[17]
0 : eject,
1 : it appears to disappear,
0 : the face flattens as it curves, curves as it flattens in
unification,[18]
1 : desire,

1 : it folds back to desire,
0 : spiral back,

1. "But this fault, this deficiency, this '***hole***,' inevitably affords woman too few figurations, images, or representations by which to represent herself. It is not that she lacks some 'master signifier' or that none is imposed upon her, but rather that access to a signifying economy, to the coining of signifiers, is difficult or even impossible for her because she remains an outsider, herself (a) subject to their norms." Luce Irigaray, *Speculum of the Other Woman* (1974; Ithaca, NY: Cornell University Press, 1985), 71 (emphasis added).

2. "The flip side of the cyborg's violation of boundaries is what Haraway calls its 'pleasurably tight coupling' between ***parts*** that are not supposed to touch. Mingling erotically charged violations with potent new fusions, the cyborg becomes the stage on which are performed contestations about the body boundaries that have often marked class, ethnic, and cultural differences." N. Katherine Hayles, *How We Became Posthuman* (Chicago: University of Chicago Press, 1999), 85 (emphasis added).

   "Recursion is the movement that tirelessly integrates contingency into its own functioning to realize its telos. In so doing it generates an impenetrable complexity in the course of time. Organisms exhibit a complexity of relations between ***parts*** and whole inside the body and with its environment (e.g., structural coupling) in its functioning." Yuk Hui, *Recursivity and Contingency* (London: Rowman & Littlefield, 2019), 15 (emphasis added).

3. "She is 'not-all,' 'not-***whole***,' 'not-one,' and whatever she knows can only be described as 'not-knowledge.' [...] She has no place like home, nothing of her own, 'other than the place of the Other which,' writes Lacan, 'I designate with a capital O.'" Sadie Plant, *Zeros and Ones: Digital Women and the New Technoculture* (New York: Doubleday, 1997), 35 (emphasis added).

4. "Conjunction of the system and of its extreme alternative like the ***two sides*** of a curved mirror, a 'vicious' curvature of a political space that is henceforth magnetized, circularized, reversibilized from the right to the left, a torsion that is like that of the evil spirit

of commutation, the ***whole*** system, the infinity of capital folded back on its own surface: transfinite? And is it not the same for desire and the libidinal space? Conjunction of desire and value, of desire and capital." Jean Baudrillard, *Simulacra and Simulation* (Ann Arbor: University of Michigan Press, 1994), 18 (emphasis added).

5. "In the 'verite' experience it is not a question of secrecy or perversion, but of a sort of frisson of the real, or of an aesthetics of the hyperreal, a frisson of vertiginous and phony exactitude, a frisson of simultaneous distancing and magnification, of distortion of scale, of an excessive ***transparency***." Ibid., 28 (emphasis added).

6. "I will call those texts in which the displacement is most apparent *information narratives*. [...] One could focus on ***pattern*** in any era, but the peculiarity of ***pattern*** in these texts is its interpenetration with randomness and its implicit challenge to physicality. ***Pattern*** *tends to overwhelm presence*, leading to a construction of immateriality that depends not on spirituality or even consciousness but only on information." Hayles, 35 (some emphasis added).

   "Randomness tears holes in ***pattern***, allowing the white noise of the background to pour through." Ibid., 248 (emphasis added).

   "[...] the interplay between absence and ***pattern*** can be called, following Jean Baudrillard, hyperreality." Ibid., 249 (emphasis added).

7. "[Psychoanalysis] even found new ways of inscribing in ***desire*** the negative law of lack, the external rule of pleasure, and the transcendent ideal of phantasy." Gilles Deleuze and Félix Guattari, *A Thousand Plateaus* (1980; Minneapolis: University of Minnesota Press, 1987), 155 (emphasis added).

   "[The body without organs] is the plane of consistency or the field of immanence of ***desire***. Even when it falls into the void of too-sudden destratification, or into the proliferation of a cancerous stratum, it is still ***desire***. ***Desire*** stretches that far: desiring one's own annihilation, or desiring the power to annihilate. Money, army, police, and State ***desire***, fascist ***desire***, even fascism is ***desire***." Ibid., 165 (emphasis added).

"To be constituted by another's ***desire*** is not the same thing as to be alienated in the violent separation of the labourer from his product." Donna J. Haraway, *Simians, Cyborgs, and Women: The Reinvention of Nature* (New York: Routledge, 1991), 159 (emphasis added).

8. "***Information***, which is neither energy nor matter, demands a new place in ontology and reconstitutes the relations between other categories, as well as the foundations of knowledge, just as Bateson and Simondon did by bringing information together with recursion. It reacts against the tendency of separating active form from inert matter in classical metaphysics [...]." Hui, 148 (emphasis added).

9. "[Carl] Freedman points out that the schizophrenic subject, as theorized by Lacan, Deleuze, Guattari, and others, evolves as an interplay between an ***alienated*** 'I' and an alienating 'not I.'" Hayles, 167 (emphasis added).

10. "The Chthulucene does not close in on itself; it does not round off; its contact zones are ubiquitous and continuously spin out ***loopy*** tendrils. Spider is a much better future for sympoiesis than any inadequately leggy vertebrate of whatever pantheon. Tentacularity is symchthonic, wound with abyssal and dreadful graspings, frayings, and weavings, passing relays again and again, in the generative recursions that make up living and dying." Donna J. Haraway, *Staying with the Trouble* (Durham, NC: Duke University Press, 2016), 33 (emphasis added).

11. "[...] the ***zeros and ones*** of machine code do far more than hark back to the binaries their logical symbols represent. [...] In both

electronic systems and the punched cards of weaving machines, a hole is one, and a blank is zero, in which case there are two missing elements, if missing is where either can be said to go. No longer a world of ones and not-ones, or something and nothing, thing and gap, but rather not-holes and holes, not-nothing and nothing, gap and not-gap." Plant, 56–57 (emphasis added).

"If we can capture the Form of ***ones and zeros*** in a nonbiological medium—say, on a computer disk—why do we need the body's superfluous flesh?" Hayles, 13 (emphasis added).

12. "[...] ***simulation*** threatens the difference between the 'true' and the 'false,' the 'real' and the 'imaginary.'" Baudrillard, 3 (emphasis added).

    In the short stories of Philip K. Dick, "one is from the start in a total ***simulation***, without origin, immanent, without a past, without a future, a diffusion of all coordinates (mental, temporal, spatial, signaletic)—it is not about a parallel universe, a double universe, or even a possible universe—neither possible, impossible, neither real nor unreal: *hyperreal*—it is a universe of ***simulation***, which is something else altogether." Ibid., 125 (some emphasis added).

13. "[...] if it is practically impossible to isolate the process of simulation, through the force of inertia of the ***real*** that surrounds us, the opposite is also true (and this reversibility itself is part of the apparatus of simulation and the impotence of power): namely, it is now *impossible to isolate the process of the* ***real***, or to prove the ***real***." Ibid., 21 (some emphasis added).

14. "[...] there is an organic ***whole*** between the individual and the collective that cannot be separated like fish and water; this organic part-whole relation is the condition of the theory of individuation." Hui, 194 (emphasis added).

15. "The everydayness of the terrestrial habitat itself elevated to the

rank of cosmic value, hypostatized in space—the satellization of the real in the transcendence of space—it is the end of metaphysics, the end of the phantasm, the end of science fiction—the era of ***hyperreality*** begins." Baudrillard, 124 (emphasis added).

16. "[…] cybernetic machines are acquiring a kind of organicity, thus becoming the ***organizing*** *inorganic*." Hui, 29 (some emphasis added).

17. "Organology signifies a shift from one recursive form (in nature) to another. It is a synthetic thought that not only integrates but also searches for a new epistemology that creates a new loop. Georges Canguilhem was the first, as far as we know, to propose the term *general organology* in order to rethink the relation between ***organism*** and machine, a rethinking that does not take the machine as the equivalent of the human but rather thinks of the human-machine as an *organic whole*." Ibid., 25 (some emphasis added).

18. "*Cosmotechnics* means primarily the unification of moral and cosmic order through technical activities; this ***unification*** is a reattachment of the figure to the ground, but it is not a return to metaphysics of the one and the all." Ibid., 29 (some emphasis added).

Hyunjeung Kim

Free Strolling

I rush out of my house early in the morning, anxious about the unfamiliar experience that lies ahead. When I arrive at Yangdeokwon Terminal ahead of schedule, I have to wait for the Happitory officer to pick me up. I stroll the serene and quiet neighborhood, feeling like a total stranger.

I remember the news coverage of Happitory that I recently watched. It shocked me to learn that I would be staying in a place built like a prison. All I had expected was to write an essay about my feelings after spending a day isolated from the world around me.

When I finally arrive at the facility, and my room is locked from the outside, I don't feel the expected fear or dread. I receive meals through a slot at the bottom of the door, just like the one in prison. Even this feels interesting, not unsettling. Since I don't have my smartphone, I can only pray, write letters, take naps, and read books. The winter landscape, framed by my window, is a huge relief.

During a nap, I slip into unconsciousness then am suddenly roused by a realization. It has to do with a past relationship which didn't end clearly. The problems that were burdening me, and that I never took the time to understand, begin to resolve themselves. My body is lifted; my mind, liberated.

The room is approximately five meters square—not small at all. It makes me think about the many things I hold onto. Why do I need so much space and so many things to live? Is it because I cannot tolerate any discomfort? I wonder if I could live a satisfied life with only a minimum amount of space, a minimum amount of food, something to read, a view through the window, and a healthy body and soul.

I brew endless cups of yellow tea. With each sip, my entire body warms. I focus on the sound of the tea brewing, which has become the only background music in such a quiet place. When I pour, I think of nature—a murmuring stream. The experience is surreal.

In this room, I can hear the sounds that are muffled in my daily life in the city. I can finally hear my inner voice. For a long time, I was not able to recognize my feelings or tend to them. I didn't take care of myself. But here, that's happening naturally in the flow of my consciousness. I've longed for such a moment.

When I leave Happitory and return to my normal life, I believe I will know (if nothing else) how to create such an environment. And I will remember this time, when I first considered how my life might be like a prison: the place I build to justify my behavior, when I blame the people around me.

*

In the wake of the 2014 Sewol ferry disaster,[1] Korean society experienced digital solidarity that had never existed before. I witnessed it, and I saw acquaintances ending their friendships, because they had different opinions about the incident. Rather than enter the fray, I felt inclined to keep my distance as events unfolded.

I had blindly trusted the media prior to the disaster, but it seemed to have less impact on public opinion than the diverse digital platforms that were forming and consolidating. The most powerful material, with the force to cause social change, came not from the top but the bottom. I need to emphasize that the solidarity achieved through digital platforms enabled this phenomenon. It's hard to put the feeling of solidarity into one word, but 'affection' might do.

In 2018, I curated *Common Front, Affectively* at Nam June Paik Art Center, which stemmed from this feeling. I wanted the exhibition to be a common ground where diverse voices could be heard together, as if in a swarm. Conceptually, *Common Front, Affectively* was designed to reflect a number of sentiments from that time, which led to collective action in the digital network—and unexpected sociopolitical change. Thirteen artists and artist groups participated,[2] channeling the unstable and precarious flow of emotions into contemporary art.

*

> Potentiality [...] is where *some things* reside, just before, since forever and always, it or they actualize and transform into something [...] Possibility and possibilities can be produced, just use your imagination. Potentiality on the other hand can not be produced, only the production of it's [sic] possibility to occur. There are no guarantees, concerning potentiality nothing is secure, it can not be calculated, it is not a matter of probability but instead of contingency. The only thing that is necessary is that something or not will occur.[3]

When I think of my twenty-four-hour experience at Happitory as a one-person performance (which is how

Mårten Spångberg might see it),[4] I focus on my body's potentiality. I wanted to explore both my doubt and curiosity. I wondered if I could learn something about my physical and spiritual conditions that I hadn't recognized before—if I could let myself go without reasoning or calculation. Perhaps I shouldn't have set any purpose at all.

My room was like a cave, allowing me to escape the larger world and the bad luck that follows after me, like the "little hunchback" in Hannah Arendt's essay "Walter Benjamin: 1892–1940." Arendt sees this fairytale figure as a motif in Benjamin's life, which was also marked by bad luck and misfortune. Describing how he navigated the politics of the literary scene, she writes:

> He never knew how to handle such things, was never able to move among such people, not even when 'the adversities of outer life which sometimes come from all sides, like wolves' [...] had already afforded him some insight into the ways of the world. Whenever he tried to adjust and be co-operative so as to get some firm ground under his feet somehow, things were sure to go wrong.[5]

*

Now that I have returned to my daily life, I'm preparing an exhibition at Gyeonggi Museum of Modern Art, in Ansan, to commemorate the seventh anniversary of the Sewol ferry disaster. The parking lot right in front of the museum was once a memorial to the incident.[6]

Reflecting on the Sewol ferry disaster in the midst of a global pandemic has led me to think about the role of art in a time of catastrophe—and for those in need of consolation. *Common Front, Affectively* viewed digital platforms as open forums, where diverse events could occur with no definite conclusions reached. Three years later, I hope this commemorative exhibition can create a different type of public space: to remember the souls lost to catastrophe, so they will never be forgotten.

1. The Sewol ferry, which left Incheon for Jeju Island with 476 passengers—including 325 students from Danwon High School in Ansan—sank on April 16, 2014 off the coast of Jindo County, South Jeolla Province. When the Coast Guard arrived, the sailors who told everyone to "stay still" escaped and abandoned the passengers, none of whom survived. Questions persist about the cause and handling of the accident. For more information, see "세월호," Daum Encyclopedia, accessed April 12, 2021, https://100.daum.net/encyclopedia/view/47XXXXXXXXX6.

2. Most of the thirteen participants, including Yunjung Lee and Hyewon Kwon, were born in the 1970s and 1980s. Foreign artists included Ed Atkins and Cécile B. Evans, who were among forty-five contemporary artists recently highlighted by a Korean journal; Rosalind Nashashibi, nominated for the 2017 Turner Prize; and Ignas Krunglevičius, nominated for the 2010 Nam June Paik Award. In addition, new works by the Korean artists Yang Ah Ham and Minki Hing were presented.

3. Mårten Spångberg, "Post-dance, An Advocacy," in *Post-Dance*, eds. Danjel Andersson, Mette Edvardsen, Mårten Spångberg (MDT, 2017), 379–80.

4. Spångberg's writing is included in *Impossible Dance*, a book that reexamines the position of dance in contemporary art. Performing arts director Seong-Hee Kim, who created Dawon Arts Festival and built the platform for years, invited several dancers and choreographers to present their projects and theories: writing on, behind, and beyond the stage. Taken as a whole, the book presents a different approach to concepts fundamental to dance, such as choreography, audience, stage, and body language. See Seong-Hee Kim, ed., *Impossible Dance* (Seoul: Workroom Press, 2020).

5. Hannah Arendt, "Walter Benjamin: 1892–1940," in *Men in Dark Times* (New York: Harcourt, Brace & World, Inc., 1955), 162. Arendt's text was originally published on October 19, 1968 in *The*

New Yorker; it also serves as the introduction to *Illuminations*, a collection of Benjamin's essays and reflections that she edited.

6. The memorial was built here on April 29, 2014: thirteen days after the Sewol ferry disaster. From then until its closing in April 2018, 728,323 people visited the site. Ansan is currently developing a permanent memorial within the adjacent amusement park; to that end, it is creating a committee of local residents, experts, and families of the Sewol ferry victims to provide counsel in the planning. For more information, see "세월호 추모공간 정부합동분향소 4년만에 문 닫는다," 문화일보, April 7, 2018, http://www.munhwa.com/news/view.html?no=20180407MW104650908900.

Min Kyoung Lee

The Break

0

I remember a story of a prisoner who became 'enlightened.' He was supposedly innocent but sentenced for a long time. Devastated at first, he soon took it as an opportunity to meditate; with diligent and determined effort, he grew calm, confident, and joyous. Nearing the end of his term, he became almost saintly.

Just before the scheduled date, the man's release was denied for some reason, and his sentence prolonged for an indefinite amount of time. His composure vanished, and with it his saintliness. He'd broken down, completely. At a certain point, 'something' happens to him, and he once more becomes saintly. This time, he'll never lose it again.

This being a supposedly true story, I've wondered what took place in him. When I was invited to spend a day in 'prison,' I anticipated having a bit of his enlightening experience.

00

In this prison, I wasn't really locked up. I had already figured out that I could comfortably exit through the food slot when they informed me of a little coin that opened the door from the inside (in case of emergency). Once I knew I could get out of the room at any time, I was able to sit back and enjoy the mock experiment of being locked in.

The conditions at Happitory were very pleasant,

and twenty-four hours seemed rather short. I chose not to occupy this time with what were obvious activities to me, like meditating and sleeping. I didn't want my mind to go elsewhere or become unconscious. Like an anthropologist, I stayed vigilant in watching out for whatever mental and emotional states might arise. I followed my mind closely and tried not to get lost in particular things.

000

I'm reminded of something I once did in Oslo, which we called *A Park Bench Project*.[1] It was directly inspired by Eckhart Tolle's story of how he had spent two years on park benches, blissed out, following his awakening.[2]

My friend Montserrat and I tried to emulate Tolle's post-enlightenment state.[3] Each day, we sat on a park bench near a theater and practiced doing nothing. On the last day, for the performance, we placed a number of empty benches in the middle of a big hall in the theater, then sat down and invited the audience to join in "doing nothing specific." Montse sat motionlessly while I moved and fidgeted as usual. Audience members joined us on the benches or sat around the room doing all sorts of 'nothings.' Soon, it was a jovial gathering, with lots of people hanging out.

When I picture Tolle sitting on a park bench, blissed out for days and years, I imagine him not doing anything special—not even 'meditation.' Jiddu Krishnamurti talks about meditation frequently in his books, emphasizing that it's not what you do but what happens.[4] (Pretty annoying if meditation never ends up happening to you.)

I learned and practiced meditation off and on for twenty years. I mostly tried to make things happen, and a few times, things happened of their own accord.

0000

I once tried to do literally nothing during a three-month meditation retreat. I lay on my bed and kept my eyes open the whole evening. Very quickly, I discovered that I had to do something, even if that just meant shifting my posture or blinking my eyes. What caused me to constantly do something was discomfort, or 'suffering' in Buddhist terms.

Upon waking one morning, at a later point in the retreat, my mind spontaneously click-entered a state of non-doing. It had no thoughts, no feelings, no movement whatsoever while being fully conscious. Only in retrospect can I make out and describe what I experienced: my mind, locked in that state for a while, before returning to 'normal.'

I'd heard and read much about consciousness being independent of the mind, or existing beyond a particular mind and body. Now I had firsthand empirical data with which to speculate about the metaphysics of consciousness and the nature of mind.[5] This never happened to me again.

000

Even though Happitory advertised a prison experience, I realized, after some research, that the twenty-four-hour program it offers is just a short version of 'The Gateless Gate': a Buddhist monastic retreat, practiced in Korea and elsewhere, where meditators are locked in a room or house—often for months. It became clear that Happitory is as much an appropriation of the meditation retreat as of solitary confinement in prison. The ability to confuse the two, for an experienced meditator and retreat-goer like myself, made me think twice about their aims and characteristics.

The common and core feature, I would say, is the facilitation of a mental break. Both deprive their subjects of social contact and sensory stimuli, leaving them with little else than their mind. Sensory stimuli function as raw materials or building blocks for our mental worlds. They help us generate images, concepts, and stories; interpretations of phenomena; and the sense of being an identity unfolding in time. When solitary confinement and meditation retreats take all this away, people might experience changes in their perception of memories, reality, and identity. No longer will they be sure of the solidity or concreteness of the world around them, which could culminate in the eventual break or dissolution of their sense of self.

For ordinary human beings, such a break is painful and most likely traumatic—even to the point of madness or death. To the prison or meditation retreat, the goal has been attained.

00

If meditation retreats facilitate such a break, how do they bring about a breakthrough and not a breakdown of a person? Contrary to the popular conception of meditation in recent years, there exist negative and traumatic reports about the experience of retreats. I've personally known three people whose psychotic conditions worsened during their retreats or monastic lives. Sure, there are probably three hundred others who left retreats feeling much happier; the fact remains that the mind is full of negative tendencies, and crossing that minefield is no easy task.

The crucial element of meditation is that it trains people to refrain from indulging in thoughts and emotions that are negative or toxic, and at the same time, to nurture positive and loving ones. This is something that solitary confinement in prison does not provide. To give an analogy: a long fast can be a great health benefit, provided you do it safely. Otherwise, it's a great danger.

The enlightened prisoner of my earlier story should not be taken as a model. He broke through eventually but nearly broke down in the process. Even the Buddha, who went down a tough road himself, didn't recommend that others follow. Who knows? You might be one of those few tough and lucky ones. But if you're not sure, you can follow the safe and proven way. Go towards the breaking gently and kindly. Merrily, merrily, merrily.

0

It was a good time, childhood. I didn't have to make money or manage anything: home, family, or career. So simple, every day was a holiday. All I did was eat, play, listen to mom, and grow. When I think back to it, that period strikes me as almost bland.

I remember an intense feeling of being emptied out, with a tinge of joy, after long hours spent playing outdoors. And I remember the sky and clouds looking shinier. That feeling was vast and light. Vast and light—that's very much the description of meditation to me.

By the morning of my departure from Happitory, a few hours before the locked door got unlocked, it was apparent that I wasn't going to have any enlightening experience. All my vigilance and anticipation, waiting and observing dropped, and I relaxed. I was okay to kill time and read the notes and drawings, funny and (un)important, that previous guests had left behind. I added one. I let myself do whatever. Things became amusing and light, like in the days of my childhood. Down or through, no break for me this time.

1. *A Park Bench Project* was part of *Living House*, organized by Sweet & Tender Collaborations and Mia Habib at Dansens Hus, Oslo in 2009.

2. See Eckhart Tolle, *The Power of Now: A Guide to Spiritual Enlightenment* (Vancouver: Namaste Publishing, 1997).

3. Montserrat Payo, a Mexican dance artist.

4. See J. Krishnamurti, *Krishnamurti's Journal* (New York: HarperCollins, 1982).

5. Reference points include Buddhism and the Indus Valley religions.

Tyler Coburn is an artist and writer based in New York. He has presented work at the Whitney Museum of American Art, New York; Centre Pompidou, Paris; Bergen Kunsthall; Kunsthalle Wien; Hayward Gallery, London; Para Site, Hong Kong; and Art Sonje Center, Seoul. Coburn is the author of three books: *I'm that angel* (2012); *Robots Building Robots* (2013), published by the Center for Contemporary Arts Glasgow; and *Richard Roe* (2019), published by Sternberg Press. His texts have appeared in *e-flux journal*, *Frieze*, *ArtReview*, *DIS*, *Mousse*, *LEAP*, and *Rhizome*.

Kyungmook Kim is an artist who works in various formats and media including film dramas, documentaries, video art, and video installation. He debuted with the short documentary *Me and Doll-playing* in 2004 and has produced several films, including *Faceless Things* in 2005, *Stateless Things* in 2011, and *Futureless Things* in 2014. These works have been screened at the film festivals in Venice, Rotterdam, London, Vancouver, Sydney, Buenos Aires, and Hong Kong. Kim's work has been exhibited at MoMA and the New Museum, New York; Ilmin Museum of Art and Arko Art Center, Seoul; and other museums.

Jiwon Yu is a curator, writer, and translator/interpreter based in Seoul. Her practice explores such topics as labor at the intersection of the attention economy and platform capitalism; gender representation in popular media and visual culture; and materialist approaches to the curatorial. Yu was an assistant curator of the 11th

Seoul Mediacity Biennale (2019–2021). Her projects include *Your Search: On-demand Research Service* (co-curated in 2018 at DOOSAN Gallery, Seoul), *(Not) Your Typical Narcissist* (2019–ongoing, online), and *Gravity Shower* (2020–2021, Daehan Theater, Gallery N/A, Seoul).

Woochang Lee, a PhD candidate in the English Department at Seoul National University, studies fiction and intellectual history in 18th-century Britain; his doctoral thesis is on Samuel Richardson's fictions and British "early feminist" discourse. He also writes about the language of debates in contemporary South Korea. His publications include "The Origin of the 'Hell Joseon' Discourse: A Study of the Narratives of Progress and the Subjects of History in Korea, 1987–2016" (2016); "A Peculiar Journey of Korean 'East Asia' Discourses and the Crisis of 'Western Modernity': From the Theory of National Literature to Political Meritocracy, 1989–2017" (2017); "The Politics and Sub-Politics of Mad Cow Disease in South Korea" (co-authored, 2022); and the Korean translation of *What is Intellectual History?* by Richard Whatmore (2020).

Sunjin Kim is an artist and writer based in Daejeon. He holds a BFA in graphic design from Seoul National University. Kim's projects include *#FriendlyStrangers* (Gwangju Design Biennale, 2017); *Take Two*, a live podcast performance (Dove Audio & Video Festival, 2017); and *The Gohomesoldier Project* (blog, 2011).

Jaeyeon Chung received her BFA from Korea National University of Arts and her MFA from Chelsea College of Arts, London. She recently had two solo exhibitions in Seoul: *Lost Corner* in 2018 at Art Space Grove and *Lost Corner_Memory Archive* in 2019 at SeMA Storage. She has been in group exhibitions and participated in artist residencies in the United States, United Kingdom, Germany, Austria, Taiwan, and Japan. Chung's work often combines video and site-specific installation, with a current focus on issues of memory, history, collective identity, and architecture. She lives in Seoul with her husband, Russell Mason.

Russell Mason was born in Blackburn, Lancashire in the United Kingdom in 1976. He studied history in college then became an English teacher. For the past twenty-five years, Mason has taught English to foreign students at language schools and universities. He met his wife, Jaeyeon Chung, in London ten years ago and moved to South Korea four years later. Mason currently teaches academic English to freshmen at Korea University in Seoul.

InYoung Yeo is an artist based in Seoul. Her work expands from the artistic materialization of text, drawing, and installation to curatorial projects with interdisciplinary approaches to gender, AI, and urbanization: her main areas of research. Yeo explores various forms of manifestation in patterns, numbers, and dimensions based on logical structures of the human 'mind,' and coincidences in multi-dimensional time and space. Her questions emerge from researching differing micro-narratives, with a focus on the cyclical 'relation.' Yeo has put together and participated in various projects, exhibitions, residencies, talks, and workshops in Korea, Germany, and Southeast Asia, among other places.

Hyunjeung Kim is a curator interested in the evolution of media and its social consequences—especially the way people communicate. She has curated several exhibitions including *Common Front, Affectively* (2018) and *Super-spreader: Media Virus* (2015) at Nam June Paik Art Center in Yongin, South Korea. She has also taken part in Gyeonggi Artist Support Center, the Gwangju Biennale, and the Busan Biennale, among others. Kim recently prepared an exhibition of three mid-career artists, which opened in November 2021 at Gyeonggi Museum of Modern Art in Ansan, South Korea. In addition to her curatorial work, Kim continues to explore ways to share art by creating contemporary art academies and volunteer cultural education programs.

Min Kyoung Lee is a dance and performance artist working in New Zealand, Europe, and recently Korea. Her ongoing interests include dance in its experiential state, the psychological state of conversion and conviction, as well as the conditions of being an artist in contemporary life. Lee has explored different performance formats, including real-time experiments inside staged fiction-dramas; performance games in which audience members are the performers; and performative statements and texts. She is a co-founding member of *Sweet and Tender Collaborations*, an international artist network, and has received the Akademie Schloss Solitude fellowship, danceWEB scholarship, and MMCA Residency Changdong fellowship, among many others. Lee's works include *How Long It Takes to Convert Gary to Communism*; *Did She Dance on Stage*; *Say, a Chinese Opera*; *Rite of Spring*; *Art, as Necessary*; *Judson Drama (strikethrough)*; and *Journey of Three Bodies.*

KEUN YOUNG CO.

It's hard to know by what, I should know, ~~is~~ that I'm not doing anything specific. It's more like I'm jumping from one impulse to another impulse before I fulfill them.

I'm trying to stop sleeping and meditation from happening, as this is something specific, and I know how time goes in with it. Not to fall into blank or an oblivion.

I guess I'm wondering, trying, being open to a new experience of not knowing what to do, without anything to do. Since it has a restriction or a condition of me writing something for the project, I think of just writing, without stopping until I have another impulse.

I'm reminded of a project and a performance I did in Oslo, called a ~~park~~ bench project, I think. In a big room, hall, a friend of mine and I invited audience to do 'nothing specific,' and had a number of empty benches at the centre of the ~~stage~~ space, a bit like stage. And my friend and I also sat and did nothing specific. We'd been practising it for the past week on ~~a the park~~ benches in a nearby park from the theatre. It was inspired by what I read of Ekhart Tolle's story of ~~how what~~ how he spent ~~his time~~ the next two years of his life after experiencing an unexpected awakening, blissed out.

Reading the description and imagining him sitting on a park bench day in, day out for two years, blissed out, I imagine, doing nothing specific. Even the meditation was, I imagine, not a specific technique, kind with a concentration ...

It's specially moving because he vividly describes ~~how~~ what an anxious person he'd been all his life.

탈진자 수는 얼마나 늘어났을까. 얼마나 많은 사람들이 고개숙니 상태 중일까.

호텔에서 매일 원고를 쓰는 고요를 누리고 싶다는 생각을 막연히 한 적은 있는데. 학위논문 쓸 때나 나를 가둬봤지..

~~Read~~ freedom in a capsule.
one huge disposable

I'm not against it. People could really make use of this.
평소에 갖는 압박을 스스로 조절할 수 있는 나이 아니고 더 큰 누군가 구해내줘야 하는 것. 엄마였나봐 일상 밖의 유혹을 재고 들기라는. 시스템으로 시스템을 깨기
Nothingness is a luxury achieve only by bashing the existing system with another system ~~of~~ of equal, or more power.

When all responsibilities were lifted about temporarily, I ~~feel~~ fell into a deep, deep sleep. Except for only a few hours when I managed to ~~put down~~ do some writing, I was deep in sleep.

자가격리를 반기는 사람들. 하지만 실제로 그 상황이 온다면?
자가격리야말로 가장 공동체적인 행위. 신뢰를 바탕으로 하는.

Writing without reference would only reveal my own dogma.
Writing without internet could get personal, too quickly.
I need to redact so many parts already.

Rhythm in writing involves all the physical conditions and the wireless network. Writing is more like a group dance, with all the right devices and software ready to roll with me. Even the fonts and font size ~~inspires me~~ leads me to a different state of mind.

no responsibility
no choice
ultimate fantasy

Saturday

#8

- Whether intentionally or not, this emphasis on writing connects to a long history of texts produced in prison [give some examples and context — Wilde, Gramsci, Pramoedya]. I wonder if former Presidents Park and [other imprisoned one] have taken a page from Kim — if, in the coming years or decades we'll read memoirs of reform or spiritual elevation from the temptations of higher office.

[Co-Celandalrio paragraphs about Lafargue, why her text is particularly compelling to me]

- Of course, given that many writers find themselves jailed for "scandalous" and "dissident" beliefs, it should come as no surprise that a pen and paper are not always readily available. [Tell apple stories, i.e. Soda]

[...]

- I lied to you earlier, when I apologized for digressing. I wasn't sorry, and in fact, I hadn't digressed at all. Everything I've said to you up until this point, was written during my period of solitary confinement. Blindness, restriction, colonialism are but facets of the experience — ways the time was passed that process reflect the influence of the setting. It would be misguided to call this writing a liberty or unburdening, because I continue to be painfully aware that this "prison" is a metaphor and a voluntary retreat. It is a privilege for a person like me to enter this prison. I can exit with the ease of a panic button.
- This is not to say that I doubt the sincerity of the facility's founders, one of them, Ms. Noh, has done drama therapy with prisoners and her sensitivity to other marginalized communities for much of her waking life, led her to recently conduct the shortcomings of incarceration a session at Happiness for juvenile offenders and their families, a wrenching [whatever the term I'm looking for... something like "prisoner reform"?] attempt to dig beneath the symptoms.
- When Happiness first opened in 2013, the main program it offered was called "Prison Inside Me." It soon came to realize that the name scared off potential clients. "Prison Inside Me" thus became [i.e.] and [i.e.], softening a metaphor still unavoidable in the facility's design.

라 같은 보슬이 남긴 51개의 수형기록 책장이다. 그들을 통해 나는 연결되어 있음을 느꼈고, 나의 상황이 최악이 아님을, 이 오늘 밤이 끝나리란 걸 배울 수 있었다. 독방에서 나의 청년을 지켜주신 분이다. 만나 본 적이 없음에도 그리운 사람이다. 21세기의 양심수, 양심들.

20세기에는 고뇌, 수치, 그리고 양심이라는 말이 있었다.

21세기에는 그 말이 관심, 영향, 자기애로 바뀌었다. 편집증적이고 나르시시즘적인 시대로 변화된 것이다.

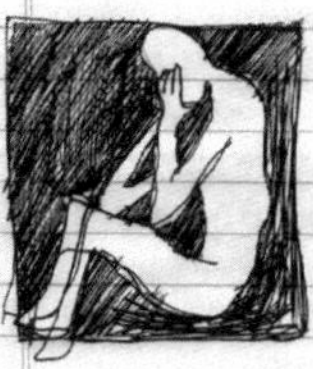

"오늘은 다만, 내일을 기다리는 날이다.
오늘은 어제의 내일이며
내일은 또 내일의 오늘일 뿐이라."

「오전 9시」

이제 곧 프로그램이 끝날 시간이다. 역시 하루는 금방 가는구나. 감옥에서도 흘려보낼 시간이 오래이 줄 건 같지 않아 시계의 초가 흐르는 시간마저도 감각할 수 있었는데 말이다. 이제 방 청소하던 숙기 쓰고 나갈 준비를 해야겠다.

예술은 세계에 의해 제약되는가? (폴 리쾨르).
〃 세계의 파생상품인가?

느슨한 인과를 갖지만 결국 거시적으로 세상에 동반되는가? (동조)

(Wag the dog)

좋다....

진문이 아니라 해석에 ... 들어가야 ??

예술은 무방비 상태로 변해가는 것인가?

Crypto, Deepfake........
예술가는 무방비 세계를 따라잡느라 급한 것 같은데?
이건 길한가?

예술의 중력은 세상의 중력을 거스를 수 있나?
세상의 질량이 더 크지?

본 풍 천

괘사!
조금씩 축적
서쪽 구름이 빽빽
아직 비는 오지 않는다

예술은 자산의 버블에 대해 면역이 있나?

예술의 내재가치가 Crash로부터 예술을 지켜줄 것이냐는 거지

예술은 CRASH 버리이었나 Asset인가?

본괘 지괘
천 수 / 지 풍

천수송 (4효)

다투려다
다툴 수 없어.
돌아와 명에 순응하고
자세를 바꾼다.
길하다.
타협의 이미지.

세상은 빠르게 변.
예술은 속도 맞추기 중요하다
버거워

본 지
산 수 / 지 뢰

어리석음을 깨우치게 하다

초효 (1효)

⑧ "EARTH IS FLAT"

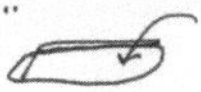

"THE SURFACE"

THE FLAT HOLE BEGIN TO END, AND AT A DOT, PIXELIZED INTO PLANETS. 7 PLANETS ABOVE YOU BEGIN TO PORTRUDE, EVENTUALLY THEY BECAME 3 DIMENSIONAL BALLS. ONE PART ROTATED, TWO BALLS ROTATED EACH OTHER, THREE, FOUR, FIVE, SIX AND SEVEN. ROTATING WITHIN ONESELF. AND EACH OTHER. THE ROTATION CHANGED ITS COURSE ITS PATH A MILLIMETER AT THE NEW BEGINNING, I THINK I'M ROTATING AT SOME POINT. WHERE IS THIS POINT IN TIME & SPACE? PART, WHOLE, ACROSS IT MEASURES THE SAME AS THE VERTICAL TIP TO TIP, HORIZONTAL TIP TO TIP. THE WHOLE COUNT OF HOLES COMES TO 14 HOLES IN PARTS, (3.1.2.1), (1;1,2,1). ONE PART BROKE, ONE PART BECAME STRONG, PARTS PARTS PARTS, FALLING INTO HOLES UNTIL THEY BECAME A WHOLE, A BIG FLAT HOLE

. . . . — – – . . .

SURFACE IS FLAT, SURFACE CURVES, BENDS FOLDS INTO DIFFERENT SHAPES COINCIDENCES EVENT.

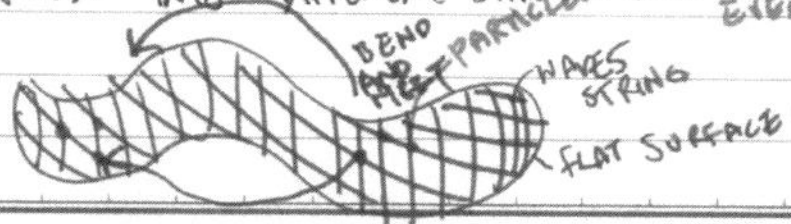

CAVE PAINTINGS? MORE ADVANCED THAN WE THINK, 3D DIMENSIONAL PAINTINGS.

독방

타일러 코번

저는 스스로를 감옥에 가두기 위해 한국에 갔습니다.

자칫 오해를 불러일으킬 소지가 있으니, 다시 설명을 시작해 보겠습니다.

2013년, 서울 동부로부터 한 시간 거리인 홍천의 산속에 한 수련원이 지어졌습니다. 사방의 전망이 탁 트여 숲이 잘 보이는 곳이지요.

'행복'과 '공장'의 합성어인 '행복공장'이라는 기관이 이 곳을 운영합니다. 행복공장은 바쁜 일상을 벗어나 스스로를 다시 돌아보고자 하는 이들을 위한 곳입니다. 이를 위해, 총 28명의 인원이 교도소 형태로 설계된 이 수련원에 머무를 수 있죠. 행복공장은 청소년, 회사원, 공무원 및 일반 대중에게 수행 프로그램을 제공합니다. 일부 세션은 연극치료를 포함하고 있으며, 어떤 프로그램은 스님이 주도하기도 합니다. 그 중 가장 흥미로운 것은 '독방 24시간'입니다. 이 프로그램의 참여자는 독방에 갇힌 채 전자기기 없이 24시간을 보내게 됩니다.

저는 행복공장이 처음 문을 열었을 때부터 이곳에 대해 알고 있었습니다. 그런 뒤 2019년 7월이 되어서야 실제로 가볼 기회를 얻게 되었죠. 다음 몇 장에서는 저의 '독방 체험'에 대해 이야기를 하고, 이 책에 참여해준 필자들에 대해 소개하려고 합니다.

*

행복공장 운영 철학의 중심은 '내 안의 감옥'입니다. 우리 모두가 각자 일정한 제약 속에서 살고 있다는 믿음이지요. 일부는 스스로 만들어낸 것이고, 일부는 그렇지 않습니다. 대부분의 속박은 익숙한 것이 되고, 의식적으로는 거의 인지되지 않습니다. 그러한 구속 속에서 우리는 삶을 만들어가고 있습니다. 우리는 이 강력한 속박에 스스로를 맞춰 나갑니다.

이 관점에서 본다면, 행복공장의 모의 교도소는 그다지 예외적인 공간으로 보이지 않습니다. '휴양-산업단지'에서 느껴지는 이상함보다는 낫죠. 사실, 행복공장에 도착하여 우리가 들어가게 되는 곳은 '감옥'이 아닙니다. 우리는 아마 난생 처음으로, 스스로가 이미 갇혀 있다는 것을 깨닫게 됩니다. 이곳에 머무르는 동안 우리는 각자 구체화된 스스로의 모습 속에 살고 있는 자신, 그리고 그 자신의 내면에서 지내게 됩니다. 불필요한 중복에 빠져 이중으로 갇혀 있게 되는 것이죠.

어쩌면 은유적 표현이 이렇게 한계에 다다를 때, 그건 스스로의 무게를 이기지 못해 무너질지도 모릅니다. 아마도, 감옥을 '중층결정'하는 과정을 통해 우리는 마침내 자유를 느끼게 될 겁니다.

*

제약을 통한 자유. 제가 아는 많은 이들이 여가 시간에 찾곤 하는 것이지요. 저희 아버지께서 중년이실 때 몇 번 하셨던 묵언수행이 떠오릅니다. 최근 제게 말씀해주시기로는, 하루하루 지날수록 생각의 속도가 점차 느려진다고 합니다. 생각을 언어로 전환시키는 행위에서 벗어나니, 더욱 편안한 페이스를

찾을 수 있었던 거죠.

'감각 상실 탱크'와 '무반향실(無反響室)'도 떠오릅니다. 존 케이지가 하버드대학교에서 그런 공간을 방문했다는 유명한 이야기가 있습니다. 틀림없이 그곳은 세계에서 가장 조용한 장소일 겁니다. 침묵이 존재한다는 사실을 알 수 있는 곳이죠. 하지만 그 방 안에도, 소음은 있었습니다. 케이지의 신경계 맥박, 그의 정맥과 동맥을 타고 흐르는 혈액의 움직임. 이러한 소리들은 우리의 삶 전체에 걸쳐 존재하지만, 세상의 소음에 의해 약화됩니다. 마침내 이 소리들을 들을 수 있었던 것입니다.

그의 경험에 대해 케이지는 다음과 같은 글을 남겼습니다. "내가 죽을 때까지 소리들은 존재할 것입니다. 그리고 내 죽음을 계속 따라올 거예요. 음악의 미래에 대해 두려워할 필요가 없습니다."[1]

*

우리 자신을 구속함으로써, 우리는 스스로를 자유롭게 합니다. 한층 높은 차원의 의식에 도달하게 되죠. 이 비유는 수많은 문화권에서 등장하는데, 주로 물질계에서는 시력을 잃지만 신성한 눈을 얻게 되는 맹인의 이야기로 구체화됩니다.

시각에 너무 의지하게 되면서, 철학자들이 몇 번이고 말했듯이, 우리는 눈에 보이는 모습을 진실에 버금가는 것으로 여겨 외적인 영역 안에 갇히게 될 위험에 처했습니다. 맹인의 다른 감각들은 시력이 우위에 있음을 계속 인지할까요? 아니면 시력으로부터 빼앗아온 감각을 서로 공유할까요? 저는

잘 모르겠지만, 디드로가 쓴 내용은 마음에 듭니다. 눈이 멀면, 피부는 세계가 스스로를 나타내는 거대한 캔버스가 된다는 내용이죠.[2]

보르헤스도 말년에 시력을 잃었습니다. 모순적이게도, 그가 부에노스아이레스 국립도서관장을 맡았을 시기였습니다. 책은 너무나도 많은데, 눈으로는 이들을 거의 읽을 수 없다니요! 자신의 상태에 대해 글을 쓰면서, 보르헤스는 흔히 '암흑'으로 치부되는 실명에 대한 통상적 개념을 불식시킵니다. 그는 맹인이 공허한 곳을 바라본다기보다 "모호하게 빛나며 초록빛이 감도는, 또는 푸르스름한 안개"[3]를 통해 보는 것이라고 했죠. 시각적 세계의 그림자 속에 사는 그들에게, 색과 효과는 없어지지 않고 지속됩니다.

*

행복공장 프로그램에 참가하기 몇 주 전, 저는 남자친구의 추천으로 준이치로 다니자키의 책 『그늘에 대하여』를 읽었습니다. 저는 글의 어조에 놀랐습니다. 제목으로 보아, 일본 미학에 대해 곰곰이 되새겨보는 책일 거라 생각했죠. 시작부터 화장실에 대한 내용을 몇 쪽에 걸쳐 다루는, 비난조의 디자인 논평집인 줄은 몰랐습니다. 다니자키의 취향은 전통적인 측면에 기대어 있고, 그 가격대는 그의 예산 범위를 벗어납니다. 그에게 있어 완벽한 화장실에는 "삼나무 가지로 채워진" 목재 소변기가 있고, "검게 옻칠된" 세간이 있을 겁니다.[4] 전등 아래에서 식사를 하는 건 사실상 음식을 파괴하는 일인 거죠.

다니자키의 책 제목은 집에 대한 그의 고민에서 비롯되

었습니다. 서구의 집은 빛을 최대한 받아들이기 위해 작은 지붕과 유리창으로 지어진 반면, 일본의 집은 유리가 없기 때문에 비와 바람을 막기 위해서는 파라솔과 같은 크기의 지붕이 필요합니다. 이러한 집에서, 그림자들은 쌓입니다. 마치 움푹 꺼진 피부에 살을 붙이듯이, 그들은 벽감과 모퉁이에 고색창연함을 더합니다. 다니자키에 의하면, 그림자는 "그 어떤 회화나 장식품보다도 아름답게" "신비스러움과 깊이를 살리는" 것이죠.[5]

*

제 남자친구가 저를 만나기 위해 한국에 온 적이 있었는데, 첫째 날 오후에는 경희궁에 함께 갔습니다. 서울의 다른 궁들과 같이 경희궁은 전체가 매끄럽게 하나로 이어져 있는 듯한 구조를 보입니다. 불에 타고, 분해되고, 산산조각이 났던 이곳은 불완전하게나마 새로 태어났습니다. 경희궁에 걸려 있는 현판은 1910년과 1945년 사이에 가장 큰 피해를 입었습니다. 봉제선 같은 이음새가 보인다면, 여기에서 식민 시대의 일화를 엿볼 수 있을 거예요.

경희궁을 산책하던 중에, 저는 몇 가지 의견을 들을 수 있을 거라 기대하며 『그늘에 대하여』를 다 읽었다고 말했습니다. 하지만 그는 소심한 목소리로 그 책을 읽지 않았다고 고백했습니다.

맞아요, 저는 충격을 받았습니다. 그가 제게 이 책을 권하면서 일본에서의 어린 시절을, 그리고 그의 특별한 미적 감각을 들여다볼 수 있는 창을 기꺼이 내주었다고 생각했던 것

같습니다. 이 감정을 어떻게 묘사할 수 있을까요? 글쎄요, 도널드 저드가 살던 소호의 아파트를 지날 때, 우리는 그 조각가가 낮잠을 잤을 법한 좁고 케케묵은 매트를 우연히 보았습니다. (저는 제 남자친구가 그걸 기억에 새겨두는 걸 보았습니다.) 나중에 우리가 함께 지내게 될 집으로 그가 생각하는 공간에는 먹고, 일하고, 섹스할 수 있는 큰 탁자가 하나 있을 것입니다.

*

남자친구가 한국에 오기 일주일 전, 저는 감옥 관광에 대한 책 『감옥으로의 도피』(2015)를 읽었습니다. 현장 조사 차원에서, 저자 마이클 웰치는 일제강점기 시절 가장 악명이 높았던 서대문형무소 역사관에 다녀왔습니다. 이곳에는 수감자 사진, 유물, 그리고 굉장히 색다른 '그림자 영상 체험' 시설이 있습니다. 이는 방문자들이 그들의 신체를 실루엣 형태로 스캔하여, 옆쪽의 스크린에 영사해보는 체험입니다. 영사된 실루엣은 90초 동안 일본 순사에 의해 감금, 심문, 고문 등을 겪습니다. 자신의 그림자가 고통받는 모습을 보며, 관람객은 그곳에서 일어난 잔혹 행위에 대해 깨닫게 됩니다.

남자친구가 한국을 떠나고 2주가 지났을 때, 저는 이 '그림자 영상 체험'을 하기 위해 역사관을 방문하였습니다. 하지만 이곳에서 저는 3.1절 100주년 기념 영상을 발견하게 되었죠. 작품 캡션은 영상을 본 관람객에게 "대한독립만세!"를 외쳐보라고 말합니다.

*

알아요. 주제에서 좀 벗어났네요. 저는 모의 교도소인 행복공장에서의 시간에 대해 말해야 하죠.

그럼요, 여러분께 말씀드릴 내용들이 있습니다. 저는 하루에 세 번, 감방 문의 작은 구멍을 통해 플라스틱 용기에 들어 있는 식사를 받았습니다. 오후 아홉 시 반에는 간수가 야간 점호를 하는 소리가 들렸습니다.

그 후로 몇 시간, 이곳은 괴로울 정도의 침묵에 빠졌는데 이는 딱 한 번 깨졌습니다. 소지가 금지된 스마트폰의 카카오톡 알림음에 의해서 말이죠.

아침은 새벽 여섯 시 천장 스피커로부터 들려오는 부드러운 소리와 함께 시작되었습니다. 메아리처럼 가득히 울리는 한 여성의 목소리가 저를 명상으로 인도했습니다. 그가 말을 마치자 저는 이내 다시 잠에 들었습니다. 또다시 일어났을 때 저는 그 목소리를 실제로 들었던 것인지, 아니면 꿈을 꾼 것인지 확실치 않았습니다.

독방 안에 들일 수 있는 것은 거의 없습니다. 세면도구와 잠옷은 소지가 가능하지만, 전자기기는 불가능합니다. 책도 가져갈 수 없죠. “모든 이는 한 권의 책입니다.” 24시간을 보내는 데에 필요한 읽을거리를 우리가 이미 지니고 있다는 듯이, 행복공장의 직원이 말했습니다.

독방에는 침대, 요가 매트, 전기 주전자와 다기 세트가 있었습니다. 작은 테이블 위에는 마커 펜, 공책, 메모지, 편지봉투 등이 놓여 있었죠.

공책에는 이 방에 머물렀던 수감자들의 성찰이 기록되

어 있습니다. 메모지는 편지지로도 쓰일 수 있었습니다. 가족, 친구, 심지어는 자기 자신에게 보내는 용도로요. 행복공장이 봉인된 편지들을 모아 원하는 목적지로 보내줄 겁니다.

*

(의도적이든 아니든) 이러한 물품을 제공함으로써 행복공장은 옥중기록의 역사에 다가갑니다. 오스카 와일드, 안토니오 그람시, 신영복과 같은 인물들의 발자취를 따라가면서 말이죠.

많은 이들에게 있어, 필기구는 손쉽게 구할 수 있는 것이 아니었습니다. 1963년, 마틴 루터 킹 주니어 목사는 신문지의 여백과 광고 사이에 「버밍햄 감옥에서 보내는 편지」를 썼습니다. 그가 구할 수 있었던 휴지와 냅킨에도 글을 적어 내려갔습니다. 그의 변호사와 대변인은 그를 하루 두 번 방문하여 셔츠의 단추 구멍 사이로 종이쪽지를 넣어주었습니다.

2013년, 베루즈 부차니는 이란의 언론 탄압으로부터 도피했지만 결국 마누스 섬에 무기한으로 구속되고 말았습니다. 자신의 글이 발견되어 압류될 것이 두려웠던 그는 왓츠앱 메시지로 회고록을 써서 번역가에게 보냈습니다. 부차니는 여전히 호주에 입국할 수 없었는데도, 그의 회고록 『산 외엔 친구가 없다: 마누스 수용소에서』가 2019년 빅토리아주 주총리 문학상을 수상했다는 사실은 굉장히 역설적입니다. 이듬해 그는 뉴질랜드로부터 난민 지위를 인정받았습니다.

*

김대중 전 대통령[6]이 "책을 읽기 위해 감옥에나 한 번 더 가야 할 모양"이라고 말하며 읽고 쓸 시간이 충분했던 투옥 생활을 그리워했다는 일화는 유명합니다. 구속을 통한 자유, 이 주제는 재차 나타납니다. 마르코 폴로가 훗날 작가가 된 수감자에게 자신의 여행 이야기를 했던 시기는 다름 아닌 그가 감옥에 있던 시절이었습니다. 마르키 드 사드의 유일한 다작 시기 또한 그때였습니다. (사드가 인생의 1/3 이상을 술집에서 보냈다는 사실은 언급할 만한 가치가 있죠.)

감옥은 심지어 한 번도 투옥되지 않은 작가들에게 있어 일종의 템플릿이기도 합니다. 애니 딜라드는 사무실 창문 너머의 풍경이 너무나 산만하다는 걸 깨닫고, 빈 벽을 마주하는 방향으로 책상의 위치를 바꿨죠. 그녀는 "매력적인 작업실은 피해야 한다"고 말했습니다. "풍경이 존재하지 않는 방을 원할 때, 비로소 상상력은 어둠 속에서 기억을 만날 수 있다"고도 했고요.[7]

*

제약을 통한 자유를 말하는 데 있어, 이 작문 과정이 해방감을 주는 행위라고 하는 것은 무모한 일일 거예요. 나의 경험을 실제 수감자의 경험이라고 보기엔 너무나 부족하기 때문에, 감금됨으로써 자유를 느끼게 되었다고 주장하는 것도 마찬가지로 무모하죠. 행복공장의 '감옥'에 들어가기로 결정한 건 저였어요. 저에겐 감방 안의 비상 버튼을 눌러 언제든지 나갈 수 있는 특권이 있었습니다.

그렇다고 해서 수련원을 설립하신 분들의 진심에 의구심

을 품는 건 아닙니다. 설립자 중 한 명인 노지향 선생님은 긴 시간 동안 재소자, 소외계층과 함께 연극치료를 진행해왔습니다. 노 선생님은 감옥의 시스템이 특정한 수준까지만 기능할 수 있다고 말씀하셨죠. 갱생의 과정에는 교도소에서의 시간보다 더 많은 것이 필요합니다. 이 신념을 증명하듯, 노 선생님은 행복공장에서 청소년 수감자와 가족들을 위한 여러 세션을 진행해왔습니다. 겉으로 보이는 모습의 이면을 보기 위한, 결코 쉽지 않은 시도였죠.

*

행복공장이 2013년 처음 문을 열었을 때, 중심 프로그램은 '내 안의 감옥'이었습니다. 하지만 설립자들은 얼마 지나지 않아 그 이름이 방문객들에게 겁을 준다는 사실을 깨달았습니다. 이로 인해 '내 안의 감옥'은 '행복한 성찰의 시간'이라는 표현으로 새로워졌습니다. 시설의 구조를 고려했을 때 필연적이라 할 수 있는 은유를 부드럽게 풀어낸 것이지요.

박근혜 전 대통령[8]이 구속된 직후, 행복공장은 새로운 프로그램을 통해 '감옥'이라는 단어를 다시 도입했습니다. "우리 자신과 우리 사회를 바꾸는 감옥에서의 20시간." 이는 국가와 지도자들을 되돌아보는 일이 수련원에게도 절박했음을 보여줍니다. 프로그램의 제목은 그의 죄가 어느 정도까지 우리의 책임인지도 묻는 듯합니다. 우리는 당시의 정치적 상황에 안주했던 걸까요?

이 '우리'의 범주에 저를 포함시키려는 건 아닙니다. 행복공장은 서구 언론에 상당히 많이 보도되었지만, 웹사이트는

한국어로만 되어 있어 외국인을 대상으로 하지는 않습니다. 저는 이곳이 한국인들에게는 어떻게 다가올지, 그 뉘앙스를 알 수 없습니다. 이 장소를 온전히 이해하기 위해, 저는 다른 이들의 목소리를 활용해야 했죠. 그래서 이 모의 교도소를 '글쓰기 레지던시'로 활용하는 것을 고안해보았습니다.

*

제가 직접 방문하고 난 뒤, 한국에서 활동하는 아홉 명의 동료들을 행복공장 프로그램에 초대했습니다. 저와 마찬가지로, 그곳에서 글을 쓰며 각자의 관심사와 삶의 이야기들을 '독방 체험'이라는 경험에 반영하도록 했죠. 이 책의 나머지 부분은 그들의 글로 채워져 있습니다.

김경묵은 한때 양심적 병역거부자로 수감된 적이 있습니다. 그는 약 15개월의 형기를 독방에서 보냈죠. 행복공장에서의 모의감옥 경험을 토대로, 그는 감옥 체제의 "억압적 질서"와 생존 수단으로서 구축해낸 "상상의 공간"에 대해 묘사합니다. 그에게 있어 가상세계는 "기술 없이도 창조될 수 있는 인간의 오래된 내재적 특성"입니다.

옐로우 펜 클럽의 일원으로서, 유지원은 참가자들의 관찰 기술을 연마하는 대안적 글쓰기 워크숍을 운영해 왔습니다. 이 책의 실험적 전제와도 공명하는 프로그램이죠. 그는 행복공장과 한국 청소년들이 일반적으로 참여하는 수련회 사이의 유사점을 찾아 글로 풀어냅니다. 이러한 프로그램은 "일상의 책무"를 없앤다는 점에서 "특유의 해방감"을 줍니다. 프로젝트의 두 번째 참여자로서 2020년 2월에 행복공장을 방

문했던 그의 텍스트에서 코로나 유행 상황은 중요한 역할을 합니다.

이우창의 에세이 「감옥, 고독, 그리고 '진정한 자아'」는 행복공장이 추구하는 자아탐색과 "자기를 돌보는" 철학적 전통을 비교하는 데 있어 학문적 틀을 제공합니다. 그는 한국의 민주화 운동에서 옥중서신이 지녔던 중요성을 다루며, 서구 사상과 한국 근대사를 통해 자유, 고독, 규율, 자아의 개념을 추적합니다.

김선진이 주머니에서 우연히 발견한 몇 개의 동전은 그에게 "변화가 없는 방 안에 갇혀, 변화의 책에 적힌 고대의 지혜를 소환한다"는 아이디어를 제공해주었습니다. 그의 글은 현 시대의 주제인 NFT, 전기차, 식량위기 등에 대해 일련의 질문을 펼칩니다. 극적인 효과를 위해 직원을 적대적인 인물로 보이게도 하며, 그는 행복공장에서의 경험으로 창의적 시도를 자유롭게 풀어냅니다.

독방에서 시간을 보내며, 정재연은 정지용의 시 「향수」에 곡을 붙인 노래를 불렀습니다. 중학교 시절 배웠던 노래였죠. 음정은 기억났지만, 가사는 "가물가물했고" 단어들은 "따로 놀았다"고 말합니다. 가사를 떠올리기 위해 노력하는 과정을 그려낸 그의 텍스트는 생략부호로 가득한 기억의 과정을 묘사합니다. 그는 명상하며 시간을 보내고자 했지만, 자꾸만 무언가 생각하게 되었죠.

근처 다른 방에서는 정재연의 남편 러셀 메이슨 또한 명상을 하기 위해 노력하고 있었습니다. 이 책을 위해 무언가를 써야 한다는 의무감을 느끼면서 말입니다. 그 결과는 '텍스트 안의 텍스트', 즉 세계를 아는 것의 한계에 대한 소고이자, 이

소고를 써내려 가는 것에 대한 이야기였죠. 글을 마무리하며 러셀은 그가 “수 세기 동안 서구사회를 괴롭혀 왔던 문제들을 거의 해결했다”고 우스갯소리를 합니다. 그는 재차 명상으로 돌아와 진정한 감사의 마음을 느끼게 되죠.

여인영은 자신이 “숫자, 차원, 그리고 패턴”으로 세상을 해석한다고 말했습니다. 행복공장에서 그는 벽, 창문, 천장, 조명 기구에 초점을 맞추어 이들이 “위, 아래, 주변 공간으로 확장되는” 것을 관찰했습니다. 그의 글은 이 경험에 대한 기록이자 이론적 명제로서 어떤 “새로운 감수성”이 “인간, 자연, 기술의 삼원적 관계” 내에 존재할 수 있는지 탐구합니다.[9]

김현정이 2021년 1월 행복공장을 방문했을 때, 그는 안산에 위치한 경기도미술관에서 세월호 7주기를 기리는 전시를 준비하고 있었습니다. 그의 텍스트는 그 여파로 등장한 디지털 세계에서의 연대가 어떤 형태를 지니는지 논의합니다. 또한, 팬데믹이라는 맥락 아래 재난에 대해 고찰하고, “대재앙의 시대에 위로가 필요한 사람들을 위한 예술의 역할”을 고민합니다.

이민경은 한때 “급진적 민족학” 실험을 한 적이 있습니다. 깨달음을 얻을 때까지 명상처에서 생활하고, 다시 “세속으로 돌아와 그 내용을 예술 작품으로 풀어내는 것”[10]이죠. 그가 인정하기로는, 이때의 위험이란 자기 자신이 예술가에서 탐구자로 변해버려 이 세계로 귀환하지 않게 되는 것이었습니다. 그는 우리의 세계로 돌아왔지만, 글에서는 다시금 깨달음을 탐구하고 있습니다. 행복공장이 명상처의 여러 측면을 전유한다면, 아마 깨달음을 얻을 수 있지 않을까요?

*

전체적으로 보면, 이 책은 텍스트의 모음인 동시에 장소 특정적 글쓰기의 가능성을 탐구하는 집단적 작업이라는 점에서 독특한 출판물입니다. 이는 비판적 공간 실천과 장소 특정적 미술, 특히 권미원의 "장소는 물리적, 제도적, 담론적일 수 있다"는 주장에 빚을 지고 있습니다. 감옥을 물리적이고도 제도적인 형태로 비유해내는 행복공장은 이 세 가지의 결합 위에 존재하고 있는 것이죠. 이 책에서 총 10인의 필자들은 다음과 같은 내용을 묻습니다. 체화된, 그리고 체현된 글을 통해 우리는 어떻게 이 장소를 포착해낼 수 있을까요? 행복공장은 고독과 자기성찰, 처벌과 갱생에 대해 어떤 이야기를 해야 할까요?

1. John Cage, *Silence: Lectures and Writings* (Middletown: Wesleyan University Press, 1961).

2. Denis Diderot, "Letter on the Blind for the Use of Those Who Can See" (1749) 참조.

3. Jorge Luis Borges, "Blindness" (1977).

4. Jun'ichirō Tanizaki, *In Praise of Shadows* (1933; Sedgwick, Maine: Leete's Island Books, 1977).

5. 상동.

6. 김대중(1924-2009)은 1998년부터 2003년까지 집권한 대한민국의 전 대통령이다. 그는 대통령 직책으로 선출된 최초의 진보 진영 지도자였다. 당선 전, 그는 1980년 사형선고를 받은 반체제 인사로 잘 알려져 있었다. 그의 형기는 이후 20년으로 감형되었으며, 그가 미국으로 망명한 1982년부터 1985년까지는 유예되었다. 이우창은 그의 글에서 김대중의 옥중기록을 다룬다.

7. Annie Dillard, *The Writing Life* (New York: HarperCollins Publishers, 1989).

8. 박근혜는 2013년부터 2017년까지 대한민국의 대통령이었다. 그는 부패 관련 혐의로 탄핵되어 24년형을 선고받았다.

9. 이 구절은 2021년 4월 여인영과 주고받은 이메일에서 인용한 것이다.

10. 이민경, 「예술이어야 한다면」, 『아무것도 바꾸지 마라』, 김정현 기획 (2016).

김경묵

하늘로 하늘로
가는 마음
맑은 바람
타고 가면
흰 구름
눈물 씻는다

— 김광섭, 「옥창에 기대어」

입소

나는 양심에 따른 병역거부로 2015년 1월부터 2016년 3월에 가석방이 되기까지 1년 3개월가량을 남부구치소와 통영구치소의 독방에서 지냈고, 행복공장을 통해 4년 만에 다시 독방 체험을 하게 되었다.

행복공장은 대다수의 수형시설와 마찬가지로 실제 사회와 멀리 떨어진 도시 외곽에 위치해 있다. 입소절차도 유사하다. 입소하면 사복에서 유니폼으로 갈아 입고, 자신의 방 번호가 적혀 있는 이름표를 받는다. 의도한 것인지는 모르겠으나 옷의 색깔이 실제 감옥의 춘추복과 비슷하고, 방 번호가 적혀 있는 이름표의 숫자는 수감번호를 연상시킨다. 이러한 과정은 수감자로서의 정체성을 형성하는 수형소의 중요한 초기 의례 행위이다. 수감과 동시에 수형자는 더 이상 사회가 아닌 교정시설에 귀속된 존재가 된다.

203호, 내가 입소한 행복공장의 방 번호이다. 다시 돌아

온 독방은 그리 낯설지 않았다. 1.5평의 직사각형의 공간, 밖에서 잠겨 열 수 없는 문, 배식구, 비좁은 화장실과 세면대, 변기 위의 손바닥만 한 거울, 방 안의 소형 쓰레기통과 좌식 책상까지 실제 독방의 환경과 꽤 비슷하게 갖춰져 있었다. 저녁 10시에 취침하여 오전 6시에 기상하는 하루의 일정, 한번 들어오면 프로그램이 끝나기 전까지 문 밖으로 나올 수 없다는 제약, 그 사이 할 수 있는 건 독서, 글쓰기 등 개인 활동뿐이라는 것 역시 감옥의 운영방침과 유사했다.

방에 들어와 가장 처음 한 일은 요가와 명상이었다. 수감시절 난 아침마다 요가와 명상으로 하루를 시작했다. 매일 반복됐던 그 행위는 하루를 맞이하는 의식이자 미치지 않고 제정신으로 그 시기를 버틸 수 있게 한 수련이었다. 행복공장에서도 이를 첫 일과로 선택함으로써 나는 좁은 공간에서 숨쉬고 움직이는 감각을 되찾았고, 수형자였던 과거의 자신과 만날 준비를 했다. 공간에 기억이 깃들듯 특정한 몸짓과 행위는 그에 상응하는 기억과 정체성을 소환한다.

두 세계의 독방

감옥의 독방은 단지 1.5평의 제약된 공간만을 의미하지 않는다. 이곳은 자신의 의사와는 무관하게 자유를 억압할 수 있는 법적 구속력을 지닌 체벌적 성격의 제도 공간이다. 스스로의 자유를 제약함으로써 더 큰 자유를 찾고자 하는 행복공장의 독방과는 다르다. 하루의 시간적 구성은 같으나 감옥에서는 오전 6시에 깨어나는 것이 선택이 아닌 의무이고, 그 시간

에 이유 없이 일어나지 않으면 처벌을 받는다. 취침 시간 외에는 방에서 누워 있을 수 없고, 무더운 여름에도 수감복을 벗을 수 없다. 방에서는 운동을 하는 것도, 엉덩이가 아프다고 수건을 방석으로 깔고 앉는 것도, 이유 없이 서 있는 것도 규정에 위반되는 행위이다. 이건 합의에 의한 약속이 아니라 입소하는 순간부터 따라야 하는 명령이다. 그렇지 않으면 그에 상응하는 처벌이 뒤따른다.

감옥은 규율과 그에 따른 복종이 최우선시되는 억압적 질서의 세계이다. 수형 기간 동안 좁은 공간에는 적응할 수 있었음에도 불구하고, 명령과 복종을 기반으로 하는 감옥의 제도적 구속력에는 단 하루도 익숙해질 수 없었다. 나는 본래부터 허리 통증으로 오래 앉아 있기 힘든 체질이었기에 의자나 방석 없이 강제된 좌식생활은 건강을 더욱 악화시켰다. 그러나 오랜 옥살이로 심각한 신체적 후유증을 얻은 다른 수형자에 비하면 이는 그리 대단한 질환도 아니었다.

이곳 203호에 설치된 창문의 크기는 한 벽면의 3분의 2를 차지할 만큼 널찍했고, 섬세하게 짜인 창밖의 풍경은 녹색의 푸르른 나무로 가득 차 평화롭고 고요했다. 반면 내가 실제 수형되었던 독방의 창문은 손바닥만 했고 창밖에는 같은 건물의 또 다른 벽면이 보일 뿐이었다. 감옥의 벽이 누렇고 바랜 회색톤이라면 이곳은 미술 갤러리처럼 새하얀 화이트 큐브이다.

그렇기는 해도, 행복공장에서의 경험이 실제 독방에서 경험하게 되는 것과 완전히 다르다고 할 수는 없다. 행복공장은 고요하고 평화로운 독방으로 감옥을 낭만화하지만, 감옥의 독방 또한 자기 자신과의 만남과 성찰을 하기에 적합한 명상적 공간이다. 감옥의 감시와 억압 체제의 반대편에서는 깊

은 자아성찰과 자기수련이 가능하기 때문이다.

정신의 공간

독방은 그 특성상 내면적이고 명상적인 생활을 유도한다. 오랜 시간 독방에 지내다 보면 물리적 공간이 아니라 정신적 공간에 기거하는 시간이 더 길어진다. 즉, 신체는 물질 공간에 있으나 정신이 거주하는 공간은 정신적 세계인 명상 상태에 빠져드는 것이다.

독방에서 생활하는 동안 나는 나만의 가상 세계를 통해 자유를 찾고자 했다. 나의 신체는 15개월간 좁은 독방에 갇혀 있었지만, 나의 정신은 친구와 주고받는 편지, 독서, 명상, 그리고 간밤에 꾸는 꿈 등 상상의 공간에 기거할 수 있었다. 나는 스스로 창조한 이 세계에서만 자유롭게 숨쉴 수 있었다. 수형 생활 중 억압과 구속이 강하게 느껴질 때면 더욱더 이곳에 의존하게 되었다. 그것은 폭력에 가까운 물리적 제약을 넘어서기 위한 생존의 한 방식이었다. 이 시기를 통해 '가상 세계'라는 곳이 인터넷과 같은 특정한 기술적 공간이 아니라, 최첨단의 기술 없이도 창조될 수 있는 인간의 오래된 내재적 특성임을 깨달을 수 있었다.

행복공장의 독방은 복잡한 사회생활과 인간관계에 지친 이들이 혼자만의 시간을 가지며 자기 성찰과 치유를 할 수 있도록 설계되었다. 24시간 온/오프라인으로 접속되어 있는 초연결 시대에 모든 디지털 기기를 반납하고서 독거 수련에 들어가는 디지털 디톡스 프로그램이기도 하다. 203호에는 이전

에 이곳을 방문한 이들이 쓴 방명록이 있었다. 그중 몇몇은 디지털 번아웃 상태를 경험한 이들이었다. 아래는 방명록에서 발견한 한 참가자의 글귀인데, 외부 세계를 차단함으로써 자신을 돌보게 되는 것에 대해 이야기하고 있었다. 이는 물리적 공간을 부정한 채 나 자신 안으로 들어가 이 방 밖의 세계, 즉 국가도 감옥도 실재하지 않으니 그 무엇도 내게 상처 줄 수 없다고 되뇌었던, 정신과 기억의 세계 속에서 살았던 때를 떠오르게 했다.

"저는 잠이 오지 않을 때
스스로를 어딘가에 가뒀다는
상상을 합니다.
아무도 나를 상처 줄 수 없고,
아무도 나를 찾을 수 없고,
시간조차 멈춘 곳에서 갇혀 있다.
그리고 언제든 회복되면 나갈 수 있다.
이 공간은 상징적으로 같은 조건입니다.
그래서 잠에 드나 봅니다.

"내 안의 감옥"은 언제든 숨을 수 있는
이런 공간의 상징적 실현 아닐까요?
당신은 죄를 지어 온 것도 아니고,
스스로를 지키기 위해
이곳에 왔으니"

방명록에 흔적을 남긴 이들 중에는 위의 글처럼 성인도 있었지만, 학교나 동아리에서 단체로 온 10대들도 꽤 많았다. 대다수 글의 내용은 이곳에 오게 된 계기나 방에 머물며 느낀 감상이었다. 흥미로웠던 지점은 성인과 청소년이 쓴 글쓰기의 방식이 달랐다는 것이다. 내 또래나 그 이상으로 보이는 이들의 글은 자신을 향해 있었고, 자기 반영적인 내적 독백의 일기 형식이었다. 반면 10대의 글은 이 방명록을 읽게 될 대상을 향해 쓰여 있었는데, 대화상대로 설정된 이는 자기 또래였고 글의 마지막에는 언제나 인스타그램 ID가 있었다. DM를 통해 더 많은 '썰'을 풀고 서로를 알아가자며. 청소년들에게 방명록 글쓰기란 디지털 공간에서의 삶과 이어지는 것이었으며, 타자의 존재가 매개된 활동이었다.

밤과 낮

저녁 7시 50분쯤 되니 해가 지고 어두워지기 시작했다. 입실할 때는 비가 오더니 이제 그쳤다. 비가 계속 내렸다면 운치 있게 창가를 바라보며 명상에 잠길 수 있었을 텐데 하는 아쉬움이 들었다. 대신 귀뚜라미, 개구리, 새가 지저귀는 소리에 귀를 기울였다. 습한 대기가 리버브 효과를 더했다. 숲의 소리에 취해 평온한 마음이 되었다. 취침 시간이 한참 지나도 잠이 오지 않아, 가지고 간 신영복 선생님의 저서 『감옥으로부터의 사색』을 꺼내 들었다. "오늘은 다만, 내일을 기다리는 날이다. 오늘은 어제의 내일이며 내일은 또 내일의 오늘일 뿐이다." 수감되었을 때 무수히 보고 되뇌었던 그의 글귀가 여전히 가슴

을 저민다. 신영복 선생님은 사상범이자 양심수로 1969년 수감되어 1988년 8월 15일 특별 가석방으로 출소하기까지 20년간 옥중생활을 했다. 내가 수감되어 있었던 2016년에 그의 부고 소식을 접하고 망연자실했던 때가 떠올랐다. 책을 다시 읽으니 마치 그가 여전히 옥고를 치르고 있는 듯했다. 그의 육체는 영면하였으나, 정신은 남겨진 편지와 함께 불멸할 것이다.

다음날 아침 6시가 되자 잔잔한 벨소리가 나를 깨웠다. 오르골로 연주된 영화 <이웃집 토토로>의 OST였다. 창밖에서는 여전히 새소리, 물소리, 바람소리가 들려왔다. 세계가 깨어나는 이 시간이 아름답게 느껴졌다. 동시에 '법을 지킬수록 기분이 좋다'는 법무부의 프로파간다 기상음악과 함께 아침을 맞이했던 감옥이 이곳과 얼마나 다른지 다시 한번 절감했다. 행복공장의 독방은 감옥의 독방과 달리 내게 스트레스나 불안을 주지 않았고, 오히려 평안과 고요에 젖어드는 시간을 선사했다. 외관은 감옥의 독방을 본떴지만 그곳의 억압적 규율은 없었다. 감옥의 독방에서 신체적·정신적 처벌 요소를 제거한 채, 그곳에서 얻을 수 있는 명상적 자기성찰과 같이 이상적인 면들만 남긴다면 행복공장의 독방과 같은 모습이 될 것이다.

아마 이 프로그램에 참여하는 어느 누구도 실제 감옥에 왔다는 기분을 느끼지는 않을 듯하다. 프로그램의 이름과 같이, 여기서 발견하게 되는 것은 복잡한 사회생활과 관계 속에서 형성된 '내 안의 감옥'이다. 행복공장은 우리가 사회라는 감옥에 갇혀 산다는 것을, 그리고 어쩌면 감옥이란 이 방 바깥의 세계일 수도 있다는 것을 가르쳐주는 곳이었다.

유지원

1.

"대구에서 오신 거 아니죠?"

미소 띤 얼굴로 날아온 투명한 질문이었다. 대구에서 코로나바이러스 확진자 수가 급격하게 늘고 있다는 뉴스를 보면서 홍천으로 왔다. 핸드폰을 제출하기 직전에 확인한 확진자 수는 총 364명. 이런 상황에서 여기 오기로 한 건 올바른 선택이었을까.

홍천역은 거의 비어 있었다. 그래서인지 택시에 오르자 기사는 안도하는 듯했다. 행복공장에 도착했을 때, 기사는 손님이 영 없다며 명함을 주고는 서울로 돌아갈 때 꼭 연락을 달라고 했다.

마음의 평화를 위해 열 명이 넘는 참가자가 행복공장을 찾았다는 건 꽤나 놀라운 일이었다. 행복공장에서 나눠준 옷으로 갈아입으며 내가 혹시 보균자가 아닌지, 그리고 만약 그렇다면 어떻게 될지 생각했다. 나도 모르게 바이러스를 모두에게 퍼뜨리고 있다면? 반대로 내가 여기서 바이러스를 얻어 서울로 돌아가 출근한다면? 나 때문에 미술관이 폐쇄되는 걸까? ~~웬 어시스턴트 큐레이터가 여행을 다녀오는 바람에 미술관을 닫게 되었다고 엄청나게 욕먹지 않을까?~~ 불현듯 우리가 무엇보다도 신체, 즉 바이러스를 매개하는 잠재적 숙주라는 사실이 뇌리를 스쳤다. 그렇다면 거리를 두는 것이 곧 돌봄이고, 만나지 않는 것이 이타적인 행위이다. 양성 판정을 받게 되면, 즉시 확진자 번호를 부여받는다. 그간의 동선은 모두가 열람할 수 있는 데이터베이스에 편입된다. 격리되어 현

관문조차 통과할 수 없게 되며, '몇 번째 확진자'라는 숫자로서 어디에나 존재할 것이다.

분명 몇 주 전까지만 해도 상황은 그리 심각하지 않았다. 확진자와 동선이 겹쳐 자가격리 기간 2주 동안 푹 쉬었으면 좋겠다는 농담이 쉬웠다. 하지만 이제 그 농담은 웃기지 않다. 자발적으로 격리되기 위해 이곳에 오고 나니, 행복공장의 감옥이야말로 지금 시점에 가장 고약한 농담같다.

2.

"내 안의 감옥에서 나오기"

건네받은 책자 표지에 적혀 있는 문구. 말로는 감옥이지만 관계자들은 선한 얼굴을 하고, 좋은 말만 하며, 공기가 좋은 곳으로 데려가 산책을 시키고, 건강해 보이는 음식만을 준다. ~~빨리 독방에 갇히고 싶었는데, 생각보다 오리엔테이션이 너무 길었어.~~ 이러한 친절에 걸맞게 낯선 사람과 웃으며 대화하고, 친근한 태도로 여기에 온 이유를 공유하느라 많은 에너지를 썼다. 방에 갇히자마자 피로감이 몰려왔다. 게다가 이 경험이 인생을 바꿀 정도로 나에게 무척 의미 있어야 한다는 압박을 느낀 것도 사실이다. ~~시작부터 틀어줬던 영상 때문이었겠지.~~ 게다가 촬영팀이 와 있다는 것도 긴장감을 더했다. 어느 외신에서 특파원을 보내 행복공장 1일 체험을 취재하고 있었던 것이다. 다른 참여자에게 방해가 되지 않겠다고 했으나, 지켜볼 일이다.

~~겨우 이틀 전에 이사하고 엉망인 집을 그대로 두고 와서 남편과 고양이들에게 너무 미안하네. 나를 미워하진 않았으면 좋겠는데.~~ 강력한 당위 없이는 이렇게 완전히 사라질 수 없었을 것이다. 프리랜서로 일을 해왔기 때문에, 언제나 나의 서비스를 제공할 수 있다는 태도를 유지하는 것이 수익과 직결되어 있다는 사실을 잘 알고 있다. 언젠가 연예인은 일을 하지 않고 그저 '존재'할 때에도 품위 유지비를 상당히 지출한다는 이야기를 들었다. 그와 비슷하게, 프리랜서 인력은 압박 아래서도 무너지지 않을 거라는 확신을 보여주기 위해 정신적인 비용을 지출하고 있는 셈이다. 이에 더해서 일정과 수입의 불안정성으로 인해 발생하는 일종의 버퍼 비용도 있다.

개인이 스스로 강요하는 구조를 '작은 시스템'이라고 한다면, 이를 필요로 하게 만든 사회의 구조를 '큰 시스템'이라고 볼 수 있겠다. 예를 들어, 이곳의 독방은 기존의 큰 시스템에 대항하는 또 다른 큰 시스템(임시적이기는 하지만)으로 작용하여 작은 시스템을 재조직한다. 한국에서 자란다는 것은 각종 수련회부터 캠프까지, 매년 최소 한 번의 큰 시스템을 겪는다는 것과 같다. 이러한 프로그램에서는 디지털 기기와 아끼는 옷, 액세서리, 나아가 주체성을 포기해야 한다. 이런 경험은 우리를 완전히 새로운 사람으로 거듭나게 한다는 신입사원 오리엔테이션, 종교 캠프, 명상 수련 등 각종 마조히즘적 판타지에 대한 호감과 적응력을 길러주는 데 한몫한다. 일상의 책무를 중지하거나 지워버리는 대안적 큰 시스템으로부터 오는 특유의 해방감이 있다.

10대 때는 독립적인 여성이 되기를 꿈꿨다. 하지만 20대가 되어 독립한 이래로는 수많은 변수를 조정하며 나 스스

로를 조직하는 것이 피곤해진 탓에, 주어진 의무를 포기하고 싶을 지경이었다. 벌써 감금생활을 은근히 즐기고 있는 걸 보면, 꽤 피곤했던 게 분명하다.

3.

이 작은 방에서는 딱히 할 일이 없었다. 일종의 안정감을 주는 스마트폰도, 두드릴 수 있는 노트북도, 심지어 주의를 돌릴 만한 책조차 없었다. 친절했지만 단호했던 요청대로 들고 온 소지품을 모두 맡기고 방에 들어왔다. 생각보다 꽤 많은 글을 썼으니 한숨 자도 좋겠다고 생각했다. 이불을 깔고 누웠다. 아직 대낮인데 낮잠을 잘 수 있다니 괜스레 들떴다.

이불을 얼굴 쪽으로 끌어당기다가 문득 문 쪽을 보았는데, 투명 처리된 작은 면적에 카메라 렌즈가 바짝 붙어 있었다. 외신 특파원이 지니고 있던 커다란 카메라였다. 분명히 방해하지 않을 거라고 했던 것 같은데? 문을 열고 들어오지만 않는다면 상관없다는 건가? ~~내가 카메라를 똑바로 응시하고 있는데도 그는 여전히 있었다. 뭐라도 문 쪽으로 던져버릴까? 미친 사람 같으려나?~~ 바로 항의할까 하다가, 생각만 해도 무척 피곤해져 그만두었다. 카메라에 찍히지 않게 사각지대에 몸을 붙여 누웠다.

~~요즘 자주 듣는 케이팝이 머리를 떠나지 않는다. 대체 왜?~~

~~*Fiesta* 내 맘에 태양을 꾹 삼킨 채~~
~~영원토록 뜨겁게 지지 않을게 이 모든 계절~~
~~나의 모든 계절 매일 화려한 이 축제~~
~~한 번쯤은 꼭 놀러 와 *fiesta*...~~

4.

도대체 몇 시간이나 잔 걸까?

시계를 가져올 걸 그랬다. 스마트폰이 시계와 알람을 겸하게 된 이래로 "시계방향"이라는 말은 수사에 불과하게 되었다. 방에 핸드폰을 가지고 들어올 수도 없었기 때문에 시간이 가는 걸 보지 못하고 있다. 정각마다 종이 울려 시간을 알리지만, 큰 도움이 되지는 않는다. ~~종칠 때 몇 번 치는지 세는 것이 생각보다 어렵네.~~ 시간이 사라진 이곳에서 자고 일어났다가, 다시 잠든다. 시간을 모르니 시간을 효율적으로 활용하기 위해 스스로와 싸울 필요도 없다. 답변해야 할 메일도 없고, 받아야 할 전화도 없다. 갈수록 졸리기만 하고 무엇을 써야 할지 생각이 나지 않는다. ~~그냥 심심해서 졸린 건가?~~

스마트폰을 갖게 된 이래로, 어쩔 수 없는 상황을 빼고는 늘 이어폰을 꽂고 있었다. 세상의 소음을 직면하고 싶지 않아서 더 크게 음악을 듣고, 지루한 오후 시간이 지나가길 바라며 팟캐스트를 틀어 놓는다.

어떤 면에서 무언가를 듣는다는 것은 실제로 비용을 지불하지 않더라도 일종의 소비행위가 된다. 청각적으로 집중하는 데에 내 시간을 소비하기 때문이다. 실제로 무언가를 스

트리밍하는 행위 자체가 크리에이터와 플랫폼 사업자의 수입으로 연결되고, 대다수의 콘텐츠에는 광고가 녹아 있으니 말 그대로 시간은 금(돈)이다.

소비는 사람에 대해 많은 것을 알려준다. 전적으로는 아니겠지만, 시간을 들여 소비하는 대상은 그 사람의 취향이나 정체성에 대해 소상히 밝혀준다. 이 방은 완전히 조용한 공간이다. 그렇다면 그 어떤 것도 듣지 않는 지금, 나는 아무것도 소비하지 않는 중이다. 지금 나는 무향 무취의, 자다 깨기를 반복하는 몸에 불과하다. 딱히 싫지 않다. 전혀.

5.

~~자다 깨기를 도대체 몇 번 반복했는지 모름.~~
~~더 이상 제대로 된 문장을 쓰는 것조차 x.~~
~~일기장을 가져왔으면 더 수월하게 썼을 듯.~~
~~이 종이가 너무 어색함.~~
~~너무 일기장처럼 쓰지 말 것. 느끼한 경구 모음집마냥 단상만 적지 말 것. 지금 그렇게 하고 있나?~~

어릴 때부터 지금까지 일기는 손으로 썼다. 손이 생각의 속도를 따라갈 수 없기 때문에 사실 기록은 생략한 채 감정과 인상을 압축하여 노골적으로 써 내려가는 습관이 있다. 이런 글쓰기는 편견을 날것으로 드러낼 위험을 동반한다. 난 여전히 자기검열을 하게 된다. 사적인 일기를 쓸 때도 타인이 이 글을 읽을 수 있다는 가능성을 완전히 배제할 수는 없

기 때문에…

일기를 제외하고 평소 글을 쓸 때는 모니터와 키보드, 워드프로세서나 메모장을 사용한다. 인터넷 사전은 필수. 맞춤법이나 각종 표기법을 확인하기도 하고, 가장 먼저 생각해낸 번역어가 최선의 선택일지 판단하기 위해 유의어 사전도 참조한다. 내가 인터넷에 의존하는 것은 철자나 맞춤법에 대한 기본 지식 부족 때문이 아니다. 아니, 그렇게 믿고 싶다. 나는 검색창이 글을 쓰는 내 뇌의 일부분이라고, 그리고 클라우드 저장소는 내 기억의 연장선이라고 생각해왔다. 이들 없이 글을 쓰면 어딘가 잘못된 느낌이 든다. 마치 내가 나 자신이 아닌 것처럼, 문단은커녕 문장 하나를 구성하는 데에도 고군분투하게 된다. 편집자나 옐로우 펜 클럽[1]의 친구 등 1차 독자와의 상호작용 또한 중요한 요소다.

내가 하는 많은 일 중에서 글쓰기만큼은 '내 것'이라고 의식할 때가 있다. ~~다른 때보다 필자로 참여한 프로젝트에서 좋은 대우를 받는다든지.~~ 하지만 나는 내 글조차 나만의 것이 아니라는 것, 순수하고 투명한 저자성을 주장할 수 없다는 것을 인정할 수밖에 없다. 글을 쓰는 환경, 도구, 사용하는 폰트, 분위기, 참고했던 책과 인터넷의 소스, 그날 있었던 일, 틀어놓은 사운드, 미리 받은 디렉션, 관련된 사람들의 기대치까지. 글은 결국 그 모든 것들이 함께 추는 춤이다.

6.

~~도대체 몇 시~~? 모두가 퇴실한 다음 기상했다. 문은 열렸고, 복도에는 이불이 널려 있다. 몇 시간이고 잠만 자다가 끝나다니. 평소의 디지털 자극이 차단된 후 나는 줄곧 수면 상태에 접어들었다. 그간 연결된 상태가 나를 억지로 깨어 있게 했던 걸까? 혹시 내면의 평화를 찾게 된 건가? 아니면 어떤 깨달음 같은 게 있었나? 뭘 (안) 한 거지? 아직 휴대폰을 받지 못했기 때문에 모든 감각이 둔탁하다. 서울에 무슨 일이 벌어지고 있는지, 나를 찾는 사람이 있는지, 내가 모르는 새에 단단히 잘못되어버린 일은 없는지, 누가 오늘 가장 이상한 걸 트윗했는지, 이번엔 어떤 중년 남성이 '몹쓸 짓'을 했는지, 넷플릭스에 어떤 시리즈가 새로 나왔는지. ~~아직 모른다. 알고 싶지 않은 것일지도…~~

독방

1. 옐로우 펜 클럽은 김빠빠, 루크, 총총이 모여 글을 쓰는 콜렉티브다. 2016년부터 현대미술 현장, 대중 매체, 서브컬처, 문학 등에 대해 글을 써왔다. 미술 글쓰기의 대안적 방식을 추구하기 위해 정기적인 글쓰기 워크숍과 리딩 그룹을 운영하고 있다. www.yellowpenclub.com.

이우창

「감옥, 고독, 그리고 '진정한 자아'」

1.

독방에 들어간다. 등 뒤에서 철문이 닫힌다. 방은 입구부터 맞은편의 창문이 달린 벽까지의 세로 길이가 3미터에 조금 못 미치며, 가로 길이는 약 1.8미터, 높이가 약 2.5미터의 직육면체 형태를 띠고 있다. 커튼을 사이에 둔 화장실과 통로, 그리고 아주 좁은 폭의 세면대가 차지하는 부분을 제외하면 수감자에게 실질적으로 주어진 공간은 가로세로 약 3.4제곱미터로 성인 남성이 딱 맞게 누울 수 있는 정도다. 구석에는 간단한 소지품을 수납할 수 있는 네 칸짜리 소형 서랍장이, 창틀에는 차를 끓여 마실 수 있도록 전기 주전자와 다기 세트가 놓여 있다. 세로 폭 길이가 팔 전완부 정도인 소형 탁자 위에는 끄적거릴 수 있는 간단한 필기구와 노트가 있다.

한 시간마다 짧게 울리는 종소리를 제외하면 창밖의 비바람 소리가—당시는 장마 한가운데였다—청각적 자극의 전부다. 철문 하단의 작은 구멍으로 간단한 석식이 들어올 때를 빼고는 다음 날 기상 시간까지 어떠한 간섭도 없다. 잠시 잠들었다가 깨니 해가 졌다. 불을 켜면 창문은 거울처럼 수감자 자신의 모습을 비춘다. 불을 끄면 잠시 완전한 어둠이 공간을 채웠다가, 이윽고 어둠에 익숙해진 눈이 창 바깥의 풍경을 어렴풋이 잡아낸다. 잿빛 하늘과 약간 더 짙은 빛깔의 산자락이 보인다. 한참 동안 멍하니 풍경을 보다 더는 잠이 오지 않는다는 것을 깨닫게 될 때, 비로소 이곳에 무엇이 남아있는가를 생각해보게 된다. 좁은 공간과 (바람을 따라 미세하게 흔들리는 능선 위의 나뭇가지들을 빼고는) 좀처럼 바뀌지 않는 풍경, 그리고 사회와 단절된 채 오직 기억과 의식, 신체로만 남은 나 자신,

그것이 남아 있는 전부다.

물론 '행복공장'의 목적은 삶에서 많은 것들을 제외하는, 부정적이기만 한 경험을 제공하는 것이 아니다. 행복공장에서 제안하는 갖가지 실천 및 그에 기입된 언어를 찬찬히 훑어보면, 우리는 오히려 이 '감옥'이 수감자에게 적극적인 어떤 삶의 양태를 요구하고 있음을 알아차리게 된다. 수감자들은 입소 전 명상과 좌선, 호흡, 절하는 법 등을 교육받으며, 몇 가지 물음이 적혀 있는 공책을 받고 그에 따라 자신의 인생을 정리해 보는 기회를 가진다. 중요한 것은 이처럼 스스로의 신체와 정신, 기억을 다스리고 검토하는 일련의 실천이 명확하게 특정한 지점을 향하고 있다는 사실이다. 그 지점이란 바로 '나', 자기 자신이다. 이 사실은 행복공장의 거의 모든 곳에 스며들어 있는 언어로부터 아주 명확하게 드러난다. 프로그램의 제목은 "나를 만나는 하루"이며, 수감자에게 주어지는 공책에는 "내 안의 감옥에서 나오기"라는 이름이 붙어 있다. 달리 말해, 행복공장은 우리에게 외부, 특히 사회의 요구와 차단된 공간에서 스스로를 탐색 및 기록하는, 요컨대 '진정한 자아를 찾아 회복하는' 과제를 부여한다.

누군가는 그러한 과제가 현대인에게 정말로 필요하다고 동의할 수도 있고, 다른 누군가는 그러한 과제가 우리를 자아의 안온한 감옥에 가두고 더 본질적인 문제를 보지 못하게 만든다고 비판할 수도 있다. 그러나 내가 던지고 싶은 질문은 차라리 이런 것들이다. 우리는 왜, 어떻게 진정한 자아가 존재하며 그것을 찾아야만 한다고 생각하게 되었을까? 그러한 믿음에는 어떠한 도덕적인 존재론이 전제되어 있을까? 우리는 어떤 기술에 근거하여 스스로를 질문과 탐색, 교정의 대상으로

설정하게 되었을까? 물론 이 모든 질문에 제대로 답하기란 어려운 일인만큼, 본 에세이는 훨씬 작은 목표만을 겨냥한다. 먼저 나는 이러한 자아 탐색 혹은 (미셸 푸코의 용어를 빌리자면) "자기를 돌보는" 전통 몇 가지의 일부를 살펴보겠다. 이어 행복공장의 독방생활 프로그램과 같은 '진정한 자아'의 탐색의 시도가 그러한 전통들의 연장선에서 볼 때 어떠한 의미를 가지고 있는지 고찰하고자 한다.

2.

철학적 전통에서 시작하자. 우리는 통상적으로 '철학'을 철학자가 쓴 어려운 책을 이해하는 일, 또는 인생의 '깊은' 진리를 성찰하는 저작을 접하고 감명과 교훈을 받는 일 정도로 생각한다. 그러나 서구의 고전적인 전통에서 볼 때 그러한 이해는 본래 철학이란 행위가 의미했던 바를 아주 부분적으로만 계승하고 있다. 프랑스의 고대 철학사가 피에르 아도에 따르면, 고전기부터 내려오는 전통에서 철학은 무엇보다도 특정한 삶의 방식을 지칭했다.[1] 철학자가 된다는 것, 혹은 철학을 한다는 것은 자기 자신을 보다 완전한 존재로 다듬어 만들어내기 위해 수행한다는 것이었다. 철학은 그러한 목표를 위해 필요한 다양한 기술과 지식의 집합을 의미했다.

고대 그리스와 로마 사람들은 인간이 적절한 단련을 통해 스스로의 역량을 개선하고 성장시킬 수 있으며, 스스로를 훈련시키고 지배하는 사람만이 탁월한 시민으로서 공동체의 통치를 잘 수행할 수 있다고 믿었다. 동일한 논리에 기초하여, 철

학자들 또한 철학적인 삶을 위해서는 스스로의 신체와 정신, 영혼을 올바른 방식으로—학파에 따라 무엇이 올바른 방식인지는 의견이 갈릴 수 있겠지만—단련하는 과정이 필요하다고 생각했다. 특히 스토아주의 및 플라톤주의적 전통에서 정신 훈련 과정은 다음과 같은 사항에 중점을 두었다. 철학자는 무엇보다도 자유로운 존재가 되어야 한다. (이때 자유롭다는 것은 자기 자신에 대한 지배권을 확립한 상태를 의미한다.) 철학자는 자기 자신과 세계를 더욱 잘 인식하기 위한 명상과 기억술 등의 실천을 통해 집중력을 끌어올려 현재의 순간에 집중해야 한다. 최종적으로 이들은 우주적인 원리와 하나가 되는 신비로운 상승의 순간에까지 도달하게 된다.

우리는 고전기부터 근대 초기까지 지속되었던 이러한 철학 전통에서 두 가지 특성을 찾아낼 수 있다. 첫째, 인간의 자아는 두 가지 심급으로 나뉜다. 첫 번째 자아는 두 번째 자아가 언제든 올바른 명령에 따를 수 있도록 훈련시키며, 동시에 내외의 부정적인 요소가 끼치는 영향력을 최소화하기 위해 노력한다. 자기 자신을 돌보는 과제는 단순히 지금의 자아를 올바르게 통제하기 위해서만 중요한 것이 아니라, 자신을 더 높은 영역으로 인도하는 것, 자아를 상승시키고 확장하려는 목표를 위해서도 중요한 일이다. 그런 점에서 충분히 훈련된 자아는 인간이 더 영원하고 참되며 가치 있는 세계로 들어서는 통로가 될 수 있다.

피터 브라운이 보여주었듯, 초기 기독교 시기의 교부들과 수도사들은 스스로의 신체와 영혼을 바람직한 상태로 다듬어 유지하고자 노력했다.[2] 그들은 한편으로 그리스·로마의 풍성한 지적 자원을 활용했으며, 다른 한편으로는 오리엔트의 사막지

대로부터 새로이 유입된 금욕과 고행의 유행에서도 깊은 영향을 받았다. 기독교인들은 철학적 전통의 두 가지 특성을 나름의 방향으로 발전시켰다. 예를 들어, 그들은 성욕의 테마를 발명하면서 자기 통제의 범위를 확장시켰다. 성욕은 모든 인간의 내면에 도사리고 있으며, 가장 덕성스러운 사람조차도 언제든 굴복시킬 수 있는 최강의 적수이다. 그에 대항하기 위해 인간 내면에 드리운 어두운 지점들을 쉴 틈 없이 탐색하고 '정화'하는 여러 방법이 정당화될 수 있었다.

푸코가 주장했던 바와 같이,[3] 자기 자신의 주인이 되기를 요구했던 그리스·로마적 전통과 비교할 때, 자기 자신이 아닌 신에 대한 절대적인 복종이 중요했던 기독교도들의 관점은 좀 더 타율적인 성격을 지닌다. 이러한 차이점에도 불구하고 두 경우 모두 자아의 도덕적 역량 및 그를 고양시키는 것의 가능성을 믿었으며, 무엇보다도 스스로를 더 높은 초월적인 영역과 연결시키고자 하는 열망이 있었다. 실제로 스토아주의자들을 포함한 고대인들의 철학적 저술, 그리고 홀로 감옥에 갇힌 철학자가 철학의 여신을 만나 신의 섭리를 깨닫는 인상적 구도를 제시한 6세기 철학자 보에티우스는 기독교 세계에서 광범위하게 인용되었다. 이후 스토아주의자들의 저술이 각국의 언어로 번역 및 소개된 17–18세기에도, 그들의 언어를 받아들이면서 바람직한 기독교인이 추구해야 할 삶의 모습을 그려내는 저자들을 어렵지 않게 찾아낼 수 있었다.

3.

마르쿠스 아우렐리우스 및 세네카와 같은 스토아주의 철학자들이 후대의 사고에 남긴 흔적 중 하나는 철학적 삶 혹은 자기수양에 있어 고독이 차지하는 높은 위상이다. 이러한 전통에서 고독은 한편으로 세속의 번잡스러운 사안으로부터 스스로를 분리시키는 것을 가능하게 해주었으며, 다른 한편으로는 자기 자신의 기억과 삶을 주의 깊게 들여다보고 잘못을 더욱 용이하게 교정할 수 있는 조건을 제공했다. 17세기 후반의 스토아주의자들, 예컨대 메리 처들리의 에세이를 생각해 보자. 처들리에게 고독이란 갖가지 정념으로부터 벗어나 자기수양 및 신앙의 실천에 집중할 수 있게 하는 것이었다. 이러한 믿음은 그 어느 때보다 인간의 사회적 본성이 강조된 계몽주의 시기에도 여전히 중요한 위상을 간직했다. 장-자크 루소의 미완성작 『고독한 산책자의 몽상』 또한 불의하고 어지러운 세속과 고요한 고독을 대비시키는 구도에서는 고전적인 관념을 계승하는 것이었다.

18세기 말 이래의 이른바 '낭만주의적' 문학은 고독한 자아의 형상을 서구 문화 전통에 깊이 새기는 데 커다란 기여를 했다. 내가 여기서 강조하고 싶은 것은 자아의 고독 자체가 아닌 고독한 자아가 접촉하게 되는 대상의 특이한 성격에 있다. 18세기 유럽 문화의 한 이상은 분명 '사회적인 삶', 즉 문명화된 사회 속에서 다른 사회 구성원들과 활발하게 소통하며 살아가는 삶이었다—그런 점에서 조셉 애디슨과 리처드 스틸의 『스펙테이터』, 새뮤얼 리처드슨의 서간체 소설이 전 유럽적인 인기를 끈 것은 당연하다. 하지만 우리는 18세기 유럽인들이

'문명화되지 않은' 세계, 즉 '미개한' 신세계나 자신들의 '야만적이고도' '고트적인' 과거, 그리고 인간의 흔적이 별로 닿지 않은 '자연'에 대해서도 깊은 흥미를 가졌다는 사실을 기억할 필요가 있다. 유럽 바깥을 다녀온 사람들의 여행기와 보고서는 많은 사람들에게 읽혔으며, 수천 수백 년 전 과거의 나라와 민족을 탐구하는 역사서들도 계속 출간되었다. '다른 세계'에 대한 관심은 고딕 소설과 낭만주의 작품을 포함해 다양한 형태의 문학 장르에서 재생산되었으며, 작품 속 고독한 자아와 '다른' 세계와의 마주침은 그 연장선 상에서 읽을 수 있다.

윌리엄 워즈워스의 1807년 서정시 「고독한 추수꾼」을 한 예로 들어보자. 스코틀랜드 고지대를 외로이 여행하던 화자는 어느 골짜기의 들판에서 홀로 추수를 하며 노래를 부르는 여성을 맞닥트린다. 18세기 후반 스코틀랜드 고지대는 '아직 문명화되지 않은' 인기 있는 관광지였다. 아마도 고지대인들의 언어를 몰랐을 화자는 실제 가사가 무엇을 뜻하는지 이해하려 하는 대신, 노래의 음을 들으면서 다양한 시공간적 이미지를 떠올린다. 그중에는 "아라비아의 사막"이나 "머나먼 헤브리디스 제도"처럼 (잉글랜드의 독자에게) 이국적인 장소도 있으며, "먼 옛날의 전투", "오늘날의 평범한 일거리", 그리고 "지금까지 있었던, 아마 되풀이될 / 본성적인 슬픔과 상실, 혹은 고통"에서처럼 과거에서 현재, 영원의 시간성과 결부된 것도 있다. 끝없이 이어지는 듯한 노래를 듣던 화자는 다시 발걸음을 재촉하면서, "더는 노래가 들리지 않게 된 지 한참이 지나서도 / 자신의 가슴 속에 음악을 품었다"는 진술로 시를 끝맺는다.

워즈워스의 시에서 화자는 거의 초월적인, 적어도 문명세계의 일상 저 너머에 있는 어떤 힘과 조우한다. 이로부터, 우리

는 이러한 '낭만적 경험의 구조'가 앞서 언급한 철학 또는 기독교 전통의 핵심적인 요소, 즉 자아의 상승 및 초월적인 존재와의 합일이라는 모티프를 변주하고 있음을 알아차릴 수 있다. 단지 과거의 전통에서 그러한 경험이 부단한 영적 훈련과 자기수양의 결과물이었다면, 낭만주의 텍스트에서는 자아의 고독과 이세계와의 조우가 그걸 가능하게 하는 조건으로 제시될 뿐이다.

4.

자아의 훈련과 확장에 관한 여러 문화적 코드 중 한 가지 덧붙이고 싶은 것은 바로 감옥이다. 근대의 감옥 담론 중에서 대중적으로 가장 잘 알려진 것은 역시 제러미 벤담의 파놉티콘 구상이다. 감시자는 죄수를 볼 수 있으나 그 역은 불가능한 원형 감옥의 구조는 종종 죄수를 철저히 무력화시키는 근대적 악몽의 상징으로 이해된다. 그러나 실제 벤담의 의도는 수감자의 굴복이 아니라 그를 사회와 덕성의 요구에 부응하는 존재로 완벽하게 교화할 수 있는 '학교'를 구축하는 것이었다. 파놉티콘의 감시체제는 어디까지나 재소자의 '교육'을 원활하게 수행하기 위한 한 가지 수단에 불과했으며, 공동체 생활과 노동을 통해 적절한 사회성과 근면함을 갖춘 구성원을 길러내는 것이 벤담의 본질적인 목표였다. 여기에는 18세기 계몽주의의 중요한 특징들, 즉 한편으로는 인간과 사회가 작동하는 원리들을 파악하려는 도덕철학과 역사이론의 성과가 있으며, 다른 한편으로 그러한 원리들을 활용하여 정의와 덕성에 부합하는 최선

의 결과물을 이끌어내려는 개혁적 의지가 있다.

인간 자아의 원리를 철저히 분석하고 적절한 환경의 구축을 통해 인간이 스스로를 개선할 수 있도록 촉진한다는 점에서, 벤담의 계획을 자기수양 전통에서 고도로 발전되어 나온 하나의 파생물로 이해해도 아주 틀린 것은 아니다. 감옥을 둘러싼 전통에서 내가 좀 더 초점을 맞추고 싶은 지점은 그와는 대척점에 있는 하나의 흐름, 특히 현대 한국사에서 찾아볼 수 있는 한 유형이다. 1960년대부터 1990년대 초까지 한국사회는 군사독재정권과 함께 그에 대항하는 강력하고 끈질긴 반체제 운동이 공존하는 곳이었다. 독재정권은 자신의 지배를 위협하는 이들을 결코 좌시하지 않았으며, 당시 여러 정치인과 지식인이 고문, 투옥, 연금되는 일은 일상적인 것이었다. 여기서 흥미로운 점은 투옥당한 일부 반체제 인사들이 감옥살이를 자유의 박탈이라는 수동적인 체험으로만 받아들이는 것을 넘어 자신의 자아를 성장시키고, 그 성장을 능동적인 과정으로 바꾸는 사례가 나타난다는 사실이다. 이러한 인식과 실천은 단순히 수감자와 그 동료들 사이에서만 공유되지 않았으며, 옥중서신의 출판을 통해 전국의 독자들에게 전달될 수 있었다.

한국의 옥중서신 장르 중 가장 널리 알려진 작품은 역시 김대중의 『옥중서신』(초판 1984, 이후 확장판 2009)이다. 이 책은 초판 기준으로 1980년부터 1982년까지 정권에 의해 감옥에 갇힌 김대중이 가족과 동료들에게 보낸 편지를 담고 있다. 그 인기는 군부독재를 비판하는 정치인으로서 수많은 위기와 고난을 거쳐 결국 1997년 대통령에 당선된 저자의 입지전적 이력에서만 비롯된 것이 아니었다. 서신에 언급되는 광범위한 독서 목록과 지적인 성찰은 많은 독자들에게 깊은 인상을 남겼

다. 또한, 감옥생활을 통해 대학에 버금가는 공부를 할 수 있었다는 저자 본인의 회고는 이후 정치범들에게 감옥생활이 지적 성장의 시간이 될 수 있다는 믿음을 유통시켰다. 『옥중서신』의 내용에서 흥미로운 지점은 텍스트의 상당 부분이 기독교적 언어에 할애되어 있다는 점이다. 신앙고백은 그의 서신에서 자주 반복되는 주제 중 하나이며, 김대중은 절대자를 향한 신앙 및 그와의 대화가 독방생활을 탈없이 견뎌낼 수 있게 하는 원동력이라고 쓴다. 자신의 고난이 신이 부여한 사명의 일부임을 받아들이고, 신의 의지를 실현시키기 위해 노력해야 한다는 믿음은 그에게 있어 자아의 다스림과 초월적인 심급과의 합일이 연결되어 있었음을 보여준다.

내 생각에 한국 민주화 운동의 윤리적 측면을 좀 더 잘 보여주는 예는 민족적 민중주의의 사고를 분명하게 받아들인 이들의 옥중서신이다. 1968년 통혁당 사건으로 무기징역형을 선고받아 20년간 수감되었던 신영복의 『감옥으로부터의 사색』(초판 1988)은 수려한 에세이 스타일로도 많은 사랑을 받았다. 독방생활을 하면서 신앙인이자 가장, 정치적 지도자로서 편지를 썼던 김대중과 달리, 신영복은 20대 대학강사 시절부터 투옥되어 다른 재소자들과 함께 지냈다. 그는 수감 기간 중 이들을 바라보면서 배움을 얻는 '민중적 지식인'의 정체성을 드러낸다. 한국의 민중주의는 민중을 단지 낮은 계급으로만 보는 대신 지금까지 핍박과 고난을 받아왔으면서도 특유의 건강한 힘과 덕성을 보유하여 종래에는 역사의 발전을 이끌어내는 주체로 보았다. 그러한 관점의 연장선에서 신영복은 민중을 직접 몸으로 체험하며 이해하고, 그들의 덕성을 배워 민중과의 합일 또는 연대를 지속하는 것을 지식인의 중요한 과제로 여겼

다. 그는 글의 곳곳에서 자신이 지금 바로 옆의 재소자들로부터 무엇을 배우고 있는지, 자신이 대학이라는 상층계급의 세계에서 배운 지식이 얼마나 헛되고 부족한 것인지를 반복적으로 언급한다. 이러한 감옥에서의 배움과 깨달음을 통해 그는 자기 자신을 다듬고, 계몽시켰다. 동시에, 신영복을 비롯한 민주화 운동가들은 감옥생활을 민중주의적 자기수양의 공간으로 탈바꿈시킬 수 있었다.

문익환은 민주화 운동 및 남북한 통일 운동에 헌신하였다. 반체제 활동으로 1976년 투옥된 이래 그는 10년이 넘는 기간을 감옥에서 보내야 했다. 그의 옥중서신은 기독교 사상과 민족적 민중주의, 그리고 자기수양 전통이 교차하는 매우 흥미로운 사례다. 그는 (자신의 아버지와 마찬가지로) 인간세계의 역사가 신의 뜻에 따라 전개된다고 믿는 장로교 목사였다. 그는 민족의 통일과 민중의 해방이 신의 뜻이라고 생각했기 때문에 기독교와 민족주의의 병립에 어떠한 문제도 느끼지 않았다. 투옥은 한편으로 그의 신앙을 민족주의 및 민주화운동과 일치시키도록 했다는 점에서 귀중한 가르침을 주었다. 여기에서 중요한 사실은 감옥에서의 요가 수련이 그의 깨달음에 불가결한 요소였다는 점이다. 문익환에게 요가 수련의 체험은 김대중의 기독교 신앙고백만큼이나 중요하고도 반복되는 주제로서, 신체와 정신의 합일이라는 자아의 문제와 민족적 역사의 거시적인 문제가 서로 분리된 것이 아님을 알게 해 주었다. 요가는 문자 그대로 자기수련을 통해 크고 작은 차원에 접근하는 기술이었다.

1990년대 들어 군부독재의 종식 및 민주주의적 체제의 정립과 함께 민중주의가 반체제 운동으로서 정치적인 설득력

을 점차 상실한 것은 피할 수 없는 일이었다. 오늘날에도 민중주의적 실천의 필요성을 이야기하는 사람들은 꽤나 남아 있지만, 그것이 한국의 공론장에서 진지하게 논의되는 일은 이제 거의 없다. 그럼에도 불구하고 민중주의가 단순히 정치적인 이데올로기가 아니라 때로는 거의 종교에 가까울 정도로 윤리적인 차원을 포함하고 있었다는 사실은 기억할 가치가 있다. 그러한 논리 속에서 민중은 가장 낮은 곳에 있으면서도 가장 높은 존재라는 위치를 부여받았으며, 지식인들은 도덕적이고 영적인 훈련을 통해 민중에 다가설 수 있었다. 민중주의의 자기수양적 측면은 심지어 기나긴 수감생활마저 영적 훈련의 한 과정으로 바꾸어 버릴 만큼 강력한 것이었다. 감옥을 '학교'라고 부르는 어법은 한국 사회의 민중적 정의와 연결되어 있는 마지막 정치범이 출소하면서 그 영성을 점차 상실하게 되었다.

5.

행복공장의 수감체험 프로그램의 핵심에는 전통적인 자기수양의 모델, 특히 스스로를 탐색하고 다스리는 실천이 놓여 있다. 명상과 호흡, 108배와 같은 행위가 단지 물질적인 신체의 조작이 아닌 신체를 통한 정신의 통제, 자아를 평정의 상태로 인도하는 연습임은 명확하다. 그렇다면 평온한 상태에 도달한 자아는 어디로 인도되어야 하는가? 수감자들의 자기성찰을 위해 주어지는 노트에 어떤 물음들이 제시되는지 보자. 지난 삶에서 행복 또는 불행했던 경험을 그래프화해보고, 인생에서 가장 행복/불행했던 순간을 각각 그림으로 그리고, 지금까

지 인생에서 발생한 중요한 사건들을 연령대별로 기록하라는 등의 문항은 수감자로 하여금 행복과 불행을 중심으로 스스로의 과거를 재구성해보도록, 혹은 단순화해보도록 유도한다. 대표적으로 "지금부터 1년밖에 못 산다면 제일 하고 싶은 일"을 그려보라는 요구는 가장 중요한 것, 가장 하고 싶은 것 외의 다른 요소를 모두 제거하고 오직 행복의 추구에만 집중하라는 명령과도 같다. 다음으로 각각 검사, 변호사, 판사의 입장에서 스스로의 삶을 "중간 재판"해보고, "나의 행복을 가로막는 내 안의 감옥"이 무엇인지 답해보라는 질문은 행복이라는 목표의 실현을 가로막는 요인을 스스로에게서 찾아내어 그것을 제거할 것을 지시한다. 마지막으로 미래 80대가 된 스스로의 입장에서 지금의 자신에게 편지를 쓰라는 문항은 구체화된 행복의 상을 떠올리게 한다. 요컨대 과거를 압축해서 조감하고, 불필요한 장애물을 제거하며, 어떻게 행복한 상태에 가까워질 수 있을지를 사고하라는 요구, 그것이 이 프로그램의 본질이다. '진정한 나'란 그렇게 행복을 위한 지향성만이 남은 정제된 자아를 가리킨다. 행복공장에서 감옥은 행복의 생산을 위한 장치다. 즉, 문자 그대로 '행복공장'인 것이다.

동시에 우리는 지금까지 살펴본 자기수양의 다른 전통들과 행복공장의 프로그램이 어떤 지점에서 다른지 생각해볼 수 있다. 그것이 철학적 이성이든, 신이든, 거대한 에너지가 깃든 문명 바깥의 시공간이든, 역사신학적 개념으로서의 민중이든, 과거의 전통들은 단순히 자아를 빚어내는 것을 넘어선다. 자기수양의 전통들은 단지 조금 더 나은 삶을 사는 것이 아닌, 조지 엘리엇이 『미들마치』에서 사용한 표현을 빌리자면, "자아를 넘어선 삶"[4]을 추구하고자 했다. 행복공장의 철학적 훈련

은 존재론의 차원에서든 목표의 차원에서든 이러한 영역을 남겨두지 않는다. 행복공장의 독방체험은 다른 전통에서 수단이자 매개였던 자아에 목적성을 부여한다. 즉, 자신을 다스리는 것은 자신의 행복을 위해서다.

나는 이러한 자기수양의 형식이 특별히 문제적이거나 해롭다고 평가할 생각은 전혀 없다. 오늘날의 세계, 특히나 기독교를 포함하여 그 어떤 종교도 근원적인 전통의 자리를 차지하는 데 성공하지 못한 한국 사회에서 초월성의 추구는 대체로 기괴하고 비합리적인 행위로 경멸 받을 뿐이다. 아마 이런 이유로 여기저기 파편화된 형태로 곳곳에서 번성하고 있는 자기수양 전통의 파생물들—예컨대 넷플릭스 TV 프로그램 〈투핫!〉 에 나오는 우스꽝스러운 '성장' 체험 프로그램들을 보라—또한 약간의 신비주의적인 향취를 걷어내면 자아를 돌보는 것 이상의 무언가를 말하지 않는다. 나는 단지 다음과 같은 사항이 궁금할 따름이다. 이처럼 형식이자 목적으로 설정된 비대화된 자아는 앞으로도 인간의 상승을 위한 열망을 충족시켜줄 수 있을까? 아니면 비대화된 자아의 일시적 유행 기간이 끝난 후에 우리는 초월적인 세계를 다시금 찾거나 만들어 내게 될 것인가? '역사'라는 그 어떤 개인보다도 더 거대한 존재에 한쪽 팔을 기대어 살아가는 사람으로서, 나는 어느 쪽의 결과가 나오더라도 쉽게 놀라지 않을 준비가 되어 있다.

1. Pierre Hadot, *Philosophy as a Way of Life: Spiritual Exercises from Socrates to Foucault*, trans. Michael Chase (Oxford: Blackwell, 1995) 및 *What is Ancient Philosophy?*, trans. Michael Chase (Cambridge: Harvard University Press, 2002) 참조.

2. Peter Brown, *The Body and Society: Men, Women, and Sexual Renunciation in Early Christianity*, 2nd ed. (New York: Columbia University Press, 2008) 참조.

3. Michel Foucault, *Histoire de la sexualité. IV: Les aveux de la chair*, ed. Frédéric Gros (Paris: Gallimard, 2018) 참조.

4. George Eliot, *Middlemarch* (1871; New York: W. W. Norton & Company, 2000), 3.

김선진

「독방에서 세상을 관망하다」

> 대전의 한 김치 공장 인수를 위해 닌텐도 사장과 내한한 아리스토텔레스 오나시스는 공장에 근무 중인 전직 여자 배구 선수와 사랑에 빠져 혼례 목적으로 LNG추진선을 타고 후쿠오카로 건너갔다. 결혼식은 일본의 전통 료칸에서 몽골인 기마궁수의 주례로 열렸다.

위 글은 기억을 환기하기 위한 키워드를 짜깁기해 만든 것으로, 최근 내 생각의 줄기를 전부 담고 있다. 외부 자료 반입이 허용되지 않은 독방에서 최근에 했던 주요 생각들을 하나도 빠짐없이 이어가려는 계획이었다. 그러나 독방에 입실하고 바깥에서 문이 잠기자마자 나는 그만 잠이 들고 말았다. 방 안은 고요했고, 바닥의 보일러는 빵빵하게 돌아갔다. 창밖 풍경은 지루할 정도로 아름다웠다. 변화를 지각할 수 없는 곳에서 인간은 시간의 흐름을 느낄 수 없는 법이다. 그렇게 나는 깜빡 잠이 들었다.

독방 안에는 스마트폰도, 책도 없다. 펜과 메모지뿐이었다. 말콤 엑스를 비롯, 인류의 역사에서 옥살이를 하며 현격한 지적 성장을 이루어 낸 전설적 인물들의 이야기를 어려서부터 동경해 왔다. 그렇지만 그들은 책을 읽을 수 있었고, 내겐 그런 특권이 없다. 아무런 인풋도 없이 어떠한 출력을 내놓을 수 있을까? 방 안에 비치된 싸구려 공책에 무슨 말을 적어야 할까? 내 의식의 흐름? 출력을 향상시킬 촉매가 필요하다. 무언가 걸칠 게 있어야 내 의식이 날카롭게 깨어난다.

최근에 본 유튜브 비디오에서 버크셔 헤서웨이의 찰리 멍거는 자신만의 '발상의 전환'[1] 테크닉을 자랑했었다. 그걸 내 상황에 적용해 보면 어떨까? 아무것도 없다고 느껴지는 현 상황

이 실은 그 반대라면? 궁핍이 사실은 궁핍이 아니라 막대한 자산을 깔고 앉아 있는 것이라면? 나에게 충분한 소스가 주어져 있는데도 단지 내가 깨닫지 못하고 있는 것이라면?

생각이 여기에 미치자 나는 내가 가진 게 무엇인지 꼽아보기 시작했다. 집에서 암기해 온 기억술 문장, 평생에 걸쳐 축적해 온 내 기억의 총체, 두 눈, 두 다리, 전인미답의 상태로 순결하게 지켜 온 거대한 무의식 영토, 주머니 속 신한은행 신용카드, 동전 몇 개.

동전 몇 개.

아이디어가 떠올랐다. 나는 동전을 던져 점을 쳐볼 수가 있다. 일찍이 퇴계 이황 선생은 동전으로 주역 점을 치는 방법을 정리해 둔 바 있다. 독방에 갇혀 한가로운 이때, 오늘날 세상의 가장 어려운 난제들에 대한 답을 점쳐보는 건 여러모로 유익한 일일 것이다. 될 놈은 된다더니, 나는 이미 척전법을 알고 있다. 바야흐로 안전마진 투자자로서 첫 발을 내딛던 2019년, '종목픽'을 압축하는 데 써먹으려고 겨우내 주역과 씨름한 경험이 나에겐 있는 것이다. 무엇보다 흡족한 건 이 과업의 시적인 부제가 떠올랐다는 점이었다. "변화가 없는 방 안에 갇혀, '변화의 책'[2]에 적힌 고대의 지혜를 소환한다." 이젠 확신을 가지고 간증할 수 있겠다. 찰리 멍거의 '발상의 전환'은 유효한 테크닉이다.

주역의 스승들은 정성된 마음으로 점칠 것을 강조한다. 어떤 미래를 알고 싶은지 질문을 신중하게 골라야 했다. 근래 내 구글 뉴스 피드 상단을 점하는 건 민족주의의 부상과 권위주의, 코로나 바이러스, 그리고 글로벌 패권 경쟁과 같은 이슈들이다. 뉴스 트렌드로 미루어 볼 때 우리가 알던 글로벌리즘

은 격렬한 변화를 앞둔 것으로 보인다. 이게 마땅히 내 첫 질문이 되어야 한다. 질문은 이렇다 — 글로벌리즘이 약화하고 그로 인해 자유무역이 퇴보한다면 대한민국은 식량위기를 맞게 될 것인가?

[지수사 4효] 군대를 숙영지로 물리면 무탈하리라.[3]

자유무역의 미래와 군대가 무슨 상관일까? 질문에 진심을 담기 위해 동전을 던지면서 태평양을 가로지르는 컨테이너 선단과 페루의 아보카도 농장의 이미지를 떠올렸는데, 동문서답 격의 괘를 얻게 되니 다소 황당하다. 글로벌리즘의 파국적 종말을 두려워하는 내 공포심의 반영일지도 모른다. 칼 융은 (융 역시도 주역 애호가였다) 인간의 정신과 물질 세계가 서로 절연되어 존재하는 것이 아님을 역설한 바 있다. 무의식적 사건과 물질 세계는 서로 영향을 주고받으며, 주역점을 치는 순간에도 이 같은 사태가 발생할 수 있는 것이다. 어쩌면 내 본심은 전쟁 발발 여부가 궁금했는지도 모르겠다.

리하르트 빌헬름[4]은 이 점괘를 "적군에 비해 전력이 압도적 열세라면, 일단 전략적 퇴각만이 몰살을 면하는 길이다"[5]라고 풀이한다. 점괘는 글로벌 패권을 쥐기 위해 치킨게임을 벌이고 있는 나라들에게 한발 물러설 것을 권하고 있는 것 같다. 그러나 자유무역의 미래에 대한 답으로는 어째 좀 싱겁다.

질문을 한층 구체적으로 바꿔볼까 한다 — 향후 15년 안에 우리는 (글로벌 무역의 쇠퇴로 인해) 식량위기를 맞이하게 되는가?

[중뢰진 괘사] 천둥이 쳐 우르릉대는 중에 웃고 떠들며 깔깔대도다. 천둥이 백 리를 놀라게 해도 제사 숟가락과 제삿술을 잃지 않도다.

점괘란 죄다 수수께끼 같은 경구로만 되어 있는 줄 알았는데, 예외도 있구나 싶다. 요란법석한 가운데서도 숟가락과 술을 잃지 않는다니, 이보다 명쾌할 수는 없다고 본다. 식량위기에 대해서는 당분간 걱정을 하지 않아도 될 듯하다. 흡족하므로 다음 질문으로 넘어가겠다.

다음으로 궁금한 건 전기차에 관한 것이다. 휘발유 자동차의 신차 생산을 2025–2035년 사이에 중단하겠다는 이야기가 정부, 제조사를 가리지 않고 여기저기서 들려온다. 전기자동차가 그렇게 가까이에 있나? 정말 그게 실현 가능한가?

[천지비 2효] 소인배가 힘 있는 자를 둘러싸고 받들도다. 소인은 길하고 대인은 막히나 종당에는 길하리라.

난해한 점괘다. 궁중정치나 권력투쟁의 상황을 암시하는 것 같은데, 그게 자동차 산업과는 무슨 관련일까? 여기서 말하는 '힘 있는 자', '소인배'는 누구이며 '대인'은 또 누구란 말인가? 한참을 생각한 후 내가 내린 결론은 다음과 같다 — 미국의 전기차 회사 '테슬라'가 바로 이 괘사가 가리키는 '힘 있는 자'다. 장안의 모든 자동차 부품사, 배터리 제조사, 언론인, 투자자, 비트코인 매니아들이 모두 테슬라의 수장인 일론 머스크의 트위터 피드에 들러붙어 떠받들고 있는 현재의 상황이 괘사 속 내용과 들어맞는다. 일론 머스크에 아부하는 자들이

바로 '소인배'이며, 괘사가 말하는 '대인'은 아마도 전통의 자동차 강자들—현대차, 기아차, 폭스바겐, 포드 등—을 가리키는 것 같다. 재래의 강자들은 캐파부터 공급망, 영업망까지 모든 걸 갖추고 있고 이들의 영향력은 대단히 '크다'. '대인'이라 칭하기에 부족함이 없는 것이다. 테슬라가 화려한 외양과 언술로 소인배들의 이목을 장악하고 있어 당장은 전통 강자들이 마땅히 받아야 할 관심이 막혀 있다. 주역에 따르면 이런 상황은 오래가지 않는다. 종국에는 '대인'이 응당 자신에게 와야 할 관심과 존경을 되찾게 될 것이다.

즉답을 주진 않았지만 점괘의 뉘앙스를 고려할 때, 전기차가 자동차 산업의 미래라는 점은 인정해야 할 것 같다. 그렇다면, 앞으로 기름때나 휘발유 냄새 따위와 남성미를 등치시키는 구도는 더 이상 유효하지 않다는 말일까?

> [풍산점 초효] 기러기가 물가로 날아가도다. 소자가 위태롭게 하지만 의로워 큰 허물이 없다.

철새인 기러기는 '떠남'의 이미지를 가지고 있다. 한 철 동안 보이다가도 이내 사라져버린다. 기러기는 왜 물가로 날아가는가? 긴 여행을 앞두고 최후의 사냥으로 배를 든든히 채우기 위해서가 아닐까? 기러기처럼, 휘발유 자동차도 언젠가는 우리 곁을 떠나가 버릴 것이다. '남성미=기름 냄새'의 등식은 이미 깨지고 있다.

전기차의 득세 — 그것은 장기적으로 원유 수요의 변화를 의미하는가? 중동의 산유국들은 변화를 대비해야 하나?

> [뇌화풍 4효] 풍족한 것에 장막이 드리워지니 해가 중천인데도 북두성을 볼 만큼 어둡도다. 동류의 주인을 만나게 되니 길하리라.

그다지 해석이 어려운 점괘는 아니다. 부유한 산유국의 하늘 위로 거대한 장막이 드리웠고 미래는 어두워 보인다. 그러나 주역에 따르면, 적절한 파트너십을 만들어낼 수만 있다면 이건 산유국들에 악재가 아닐 수도 있다. 자동차로 인한 석유 수요는 감소하겠지만 비행기, 선박, 탱크 쪽의 수요는 건재할 것이고 석유화학업계의 수요 또한 견고할 것이니 큰 걱정은 말라고 주역은 말하고 있다.

주제를 바꿔 이번에는 예술 세계에 관해 점을 쳐볼까 한다. 일단 떠오르는 건 'NFT'라고 불리는 대체 불가능 토큰이다. 팬데믹의 발발과 함께 내가 예술계와 거리를 두기 시작한 이래로 가장 많이 들은 단어가 아닐까 한다. 대체 불가능 토큰의 핵심은 상호 교환이 안 된다는 점에 있다. 암호화폐와 같은 블록체인 기반 기술로 설계되었지만, 토큰 간에 서로 등가교환이 불가능하여 (암호)화폐라고는 할 수 없다. 통화로서 기능하려면 더하고 빼고 곱하고 나누기 위한 기초로서의 '단위'를 가져야 한다. 모든 사람이 가진 1원이 전부 등가의 1원이어야만 교환이 성립할 텐데, 대체 불가능 토큰에는 그러한 균질한 단위가 없다. 토큰 하나하나는 고유하기 때문이다.

이 기술을 통해 예술작품을 발행하게 되면 작품에 고유의 디지털 표식이 부여되어 작품의 진품성이 인증된다는 것—특히 예술계 제도권의 중개 및 증빙 행위를 거치지 않고도 작품의 진품성이 확립되고 시장 접근 역시 가능하다는 것—이 그

간 귀가 아프도록 들어온 이야기다. 그렇다면, 대체 불가능 토큰은 예술에 있어 좋은 것인가?

> [산지박 초효] 침상의 다리를 때려 부수도다. 곧추선 것을 망가뜨리니 흉하다.

상황을 불문, 다리가 부러지는 게 좋은 일일 리 없다. 침대의 다리라고 예외는 아니어서 이 괘는 명백한 흉괘다. 침대는 휴식을 취하는 인간의 몸을 지탱하여 주고, 침대의 다리는 그러한 침대를 지탱하는 것이다. 주역은 대체 불가능 토큰이 예술을 지탱하는 기초를 파괴할 흉물이라고 말하고 있다. 대체 불가능 토큰은 예술의 근간을 파괴할 것이다.

대체 불가능 토큰에 대한 사람들의 반응은 갈린다. 작품을 현금화하여 그간의 예술교육과 방황에 들인 시간과 투자금을 회수할 기회로 느끼는 사람이 있는가 하면, 반대로 확립된 업계 질서와 기득권을 어지럽히는 위협 요소로 느끼는 측도 있다. 나의 다음 질문은 이렇다 — 듣도 보도 못한 디지털 작품이 단 몇 분 만에 수십 억 원의 호가에 낙찰되는 광기, 이 광기는 계속될 것인가?

> [산수몽 초효] 어리석은 자들을 계몽하도다. 훈육을 가하는 것이 이로우리라. 족쇄를 사용하지 않고 진행하면 상황이 어려워지리라.

시의적절하게도 굉장히 구체적인 조언이 나와주었다. 혼돈을 끊어내려면 훈육은 불가결한 일이다. 관건은 누가 누구를

훈육하는가의 문제다. 회초리를 집어 드는 건 누구일까? ‘NFT 아트’의 판매자일까? 혹은 미스터 마켓? 아니면, 기득권을 위협받고 있는 미술계 중간 상인들?

이를 둘러싼 모든 야단법석은 기존 예술제도를 우회할 수 있는 테크놀로지의 힘에서 비롯하는 것이다. 이쯤에서 내 불만 하나를 얘기해야겠다. 인류 역사의 지금 이 시기에, 구체적으로는 예술사의 지금 시점에 ‘작품의 고유성’ 주장이 득세하고 있는 현상을 나는 이해할 수가 없다. 고유성은 ‘가치’와 동의어가 아닌데 말이다. 대체 불가능 토큰이 담보하는 ‘대체 불가능성’이 정말로 가슴 뛰는 대단한 요소일까? 주역에게 묻고자 한다.

> [풍천소축 본괘] 조금씩 축적하는 이미지. 형통하리라. 서쪽에서부터 구름이 빽빽해지고 있으나 아직 비는 내리지 않는다.

이 괘를 확인하고 나는 주역의 신묘함에 놀라 정신이 아득해졌다.

“구름이 빽빽해지나, 아직 비는 내리지 않고 있다.”

우량한 정신을 가진 자라면 누구라도 이 괘에서 마르셀 뒤샹과 그의 ‘앵프라맹스’를 떠올리지 않을 수 없을 것이다. 구름이 빽빽해진다. 동시에 구름을 이루는 물방울 입자들도 점점 커지고 무거워진다. 하지만 아직 ‘비’가 시작될 임계에 이르진 못한 상태다. 그러다가 최초의 물방울이 제 무게를 견디지 못하고 땅을 향해 자유낙하를 시작하는 첫 순간이 바로 앵프라맹스적인 순간이다.

자연히 내 생각은 호르헤 루이스 보르헤스의 소설 「피에르 메나르, 돈키호테의 저자」로 이어졌다. 소설에서 피에르 메나르는 세르반테스의 돈키호테를 시대에 맞게 새롭게 쓰기 위해 갖은 노력을 들이지만 결과적으로 탄생한 원고는 세르반테스의 원작과 토씨 하나, 부호 하나에 이르기까지 똑같아 보이는 작품이었다. 그러나 지각 불가능한 차이로 인해 두 작품은 완전히 달라진다.

주역이 마르셀 뒤샹까지 암시하며 전달하고자 하는 것은 '일견 유사해 보이지만 엄연히 서로 다른 것들'[6]의 차이에 주목하라는 메시지다. 대체 불가능 토큰의 '대체 불가능성'은 복고적 코스프레의 냄새를 짙게 풍긴다. 작품의 기술적 대체 불가능성이 곧 작품의 고유성을 의미하는 것이 아닐뿐더러, 진품성 담론 자체도 시의성이 떨어진다. 구시대 담론이 첨단 블록체인 테크놀로지를 통해 부당하게 소환된 느낌이다.

여기까지 점을 친 후 나는 잠에 빠져들었다. 여덟 개의 질문을 위해 동전을 마흔 여덟 번 연속으로 던져야 했고, 단순한 동전 던지기가 아닌, 상징적으로 내 무의식의 지형지물을 더듬어 파악하는 일이었기에 무척 진이 빠졌다. 온기가 감도는 온돌 바닥과 독방의 고요한 음향 환경 또한 잠을 부추겼다.

복도에서 간수가 고함을 치는 소리에 잠을 깬 건 다음 날 아침이었다. 어느덧 퇴소할 시간이 된 것이었다. 묻고 싶은 것을 다 묻지도 못했는데 벌써 시간이 다 됐다니… 마음의 압박이 거세졌다. 잠이 덜 깬 상태였지만, 손놓고 있을 게 아니라 마지막까지 시간을 쥐어짜 보자고 생각했던 기억이 난다. 생각해 둔 질문을 모두 점쳐볼 수는 없겠지만, 어쨌든 할 수 있는 건 해봐야 했다.

시시각각 가까워지는 간수의 고함소리에 초조한 와중에도 여섯 번 더 허공을 향해 동전을 튕겼다. 마지막으로 떨어진 동전의 배치를 눈에 익히고 있던 그 순간, 굉음과 함께 독방 문을 박차고 간수가 난입했다. 그는 바닥에 널브러진 동전과 내 얼굴을 번갈아 노려보더니 고래고래 알 수 없는 말을 퍼부으며 나를 제압해 따뜻한 온돌바닥에 짓눌렀다. 내가 귀신과 도박판이라도 벌인 줄 알았나 보다. 내가 주역에게 물었던 최후의 질문은 이것이었다 — 마지막으로 예술가에게 해줄 조언이 있다면?

> [천택리 3효] 외눈박이도 잘 보고 절름발이도 잘 걸을 수 있지만 그러다 호랑이 꼬리를 밟게 되면 사람을 물어 흉하리라. 무인은 대군을 도와 일하노라.

수수께끼 같지만 풀이는 의외로 쉽다고 본다. 외눈박이에게 가장 절실한 건 무엇일까? 하나밖에 없는 눈으로 열심히, 잘 보는 일일 것이다. 절름발이가 가장 원하는 것은 무엇일까? 저는 다리에도 불구하고 똑바로 걷는 일일 게다. 무릇 절박한 사람이 자기 쓸모를 증명하려 과한 행동을 하다 보면 예상 못한 실수를 하거나 엉뚱한 사람을 화나게 할 수 있다. 이는 예술가에도 마찬가지로 적용되는 교훈이다. 예술가는 '무인이 대군을 섬기듯' 자기 한 몸보다 더 큰 대의를 위해 봉사한다는 생각을 한시도 잊어선 안 되며, 자기 역량을 과시하려는 딴 뜻을 품고 예술 실천에 임한다든지, 공동체에의 봉사를 도외시하고 예술지상주의적 태도를 취하다간 흉한 꼴을 볼 수 있다. 오천 년의 역사를 가진 점서가 하는 말이니 새겨 들어 손해볼 일은 없을 것이다.

1. 영상 링크 “Charlie Munger: The mental models I used to become successful in life,” YouTube video, 29:07, 2021년 1월 8일, https://www.youtube.com/watch?v=ZuHHmVX8a00

2. 주역(周易)에서 역(易)은 변화를 의미하며, 이는 영미권에서 흔히 “Book of Changes”라고 소개되기도 한다.

3. 본문에 제시한 모든 주역 괘사는 리차드 빌헬름의 해석과 황태연의 『실증주역』(청계, 2008)을 참조하였다.

4. 리차드 빌헬름(1873-1930)은 독일의 중국학자, 신학자, 선교사로, 서구에 처음 주역을 소개한 인물이다.

5. 리차드 빌헬름, “I Ching,” http://www2.unipr.it/~deyoung/I_Ching_Wilhelm_Translation.html.

6. 이를 가리키는 한자어로는 사이비(似而非)라는 말이 있다.

정재연

1.

중학교 때 담임이 음악 선생님이라는 이유로 반 전체가 합창 대회에 나가야 했다.
우리는 정지용의 시 「향수」에 곡을 붙인 동명의 노래를 불렀다.
합창이다 보니 뭐 하나라도 틀리면 금세 티가 났다. 그래서 가사를 참 열심히도 외웠다.
심지어 노랫말이 이미지로 떠올랐다.

행복공장에 들어와 이 노래를 몇 번이나 불렀던가.
어디 한번, 노랫말을 기억에 의존해서 써보기로 했다.

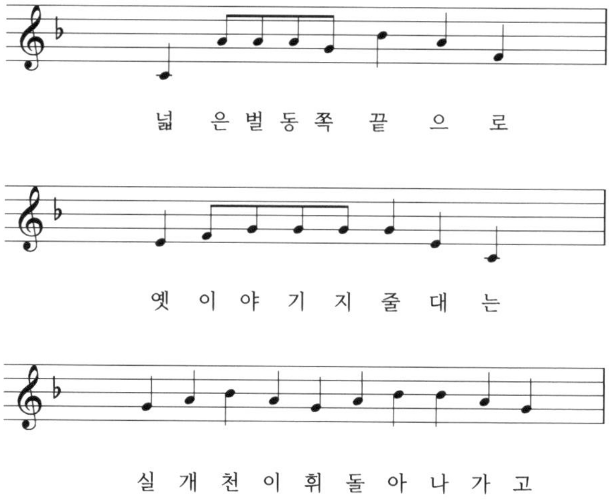
넓 은 벌 동 쪽 끝 으 로
옛 이 야 기 지 줄 대 는
실 개 천 이 휘 돌 아 나 가 고

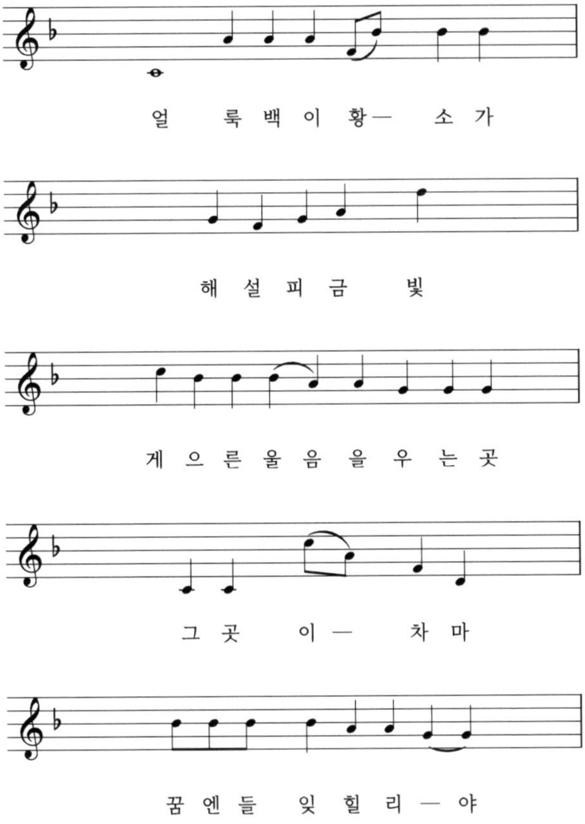
얼 룩백이 황— 소 가
해 설 피 금 빛
게 으 른 울 음 을 우 는 곳
그 곳 이 — 차 마
꿈 엔 들 잊 힐 리 — 야

역시 첫 소절은 술술 입에 붙는다.
그런데 음정만 생생할 뿐, 가사는 가물가물하다.
1절과 2절 가사들이 뒤섞여 음정과 어긋난다.
가사 내용에 치중해 불러보니 이번엔 후렴구가 어색하다.
평소 같았으면 핸드폰 검색 한 번으로 바로 찾았을 텐데…
(핸드폰은 독방에 들어오기 직전 자진 반납했다.)

나는 몇 번이고 가사를 떠올리기 위해 고군분투한다.
지금까지 나온 단어들을 조합해 마음속으로 불러본다.
마음 같아선 큰 소리로 목놓아 불러보고 싶지만,
내일 마주칠 옆방 체험자를 생각하면 후회할 게 뻔하다.
결국 나지막이 (교양을 지키는 선에서) 노래를 불러본다.

아, 그간 제자리를 찾지 못해 헤매던 단어와 음절들이 선명해지는 것 같다.
따로 놀던 단어의 조합과 서사가 조금씩 맞아 들어가는 느낌이다.

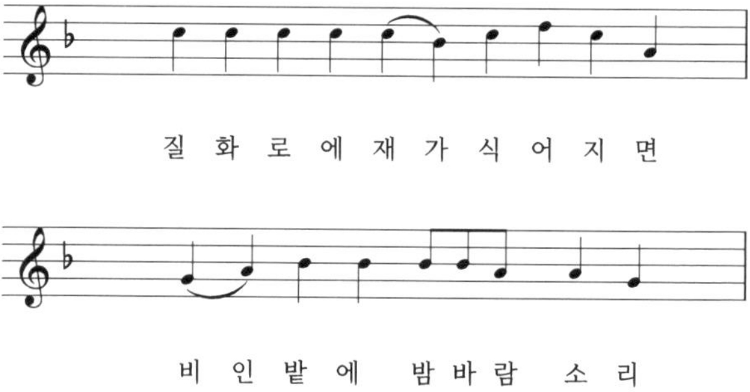

정재연

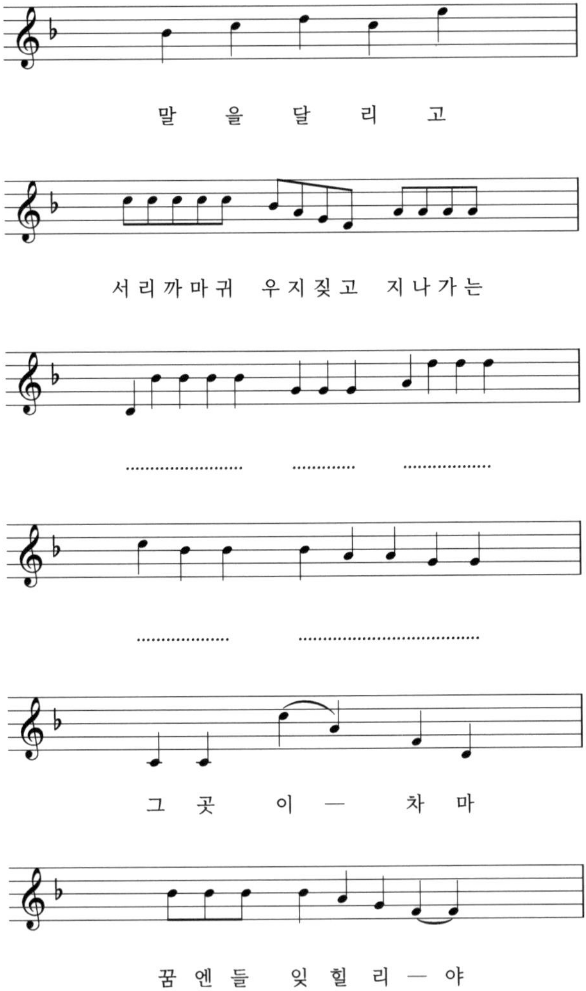

독방

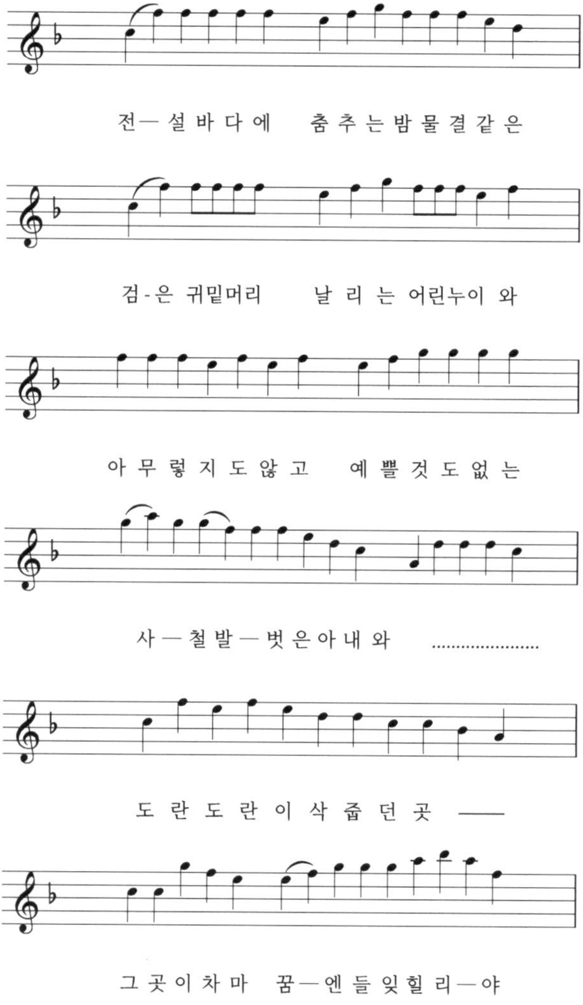
전— 설 바 다 에 춤 추 는 밤 물 결 같 은
검-은 귀밑머리 날 리 는 어린누이 와
아 무 렇 지 도 않 고 예 쁠 것 도 없 는
사 — 철 발 — 벗 은 아 내 와 ....
도 란 도 란 이 삭 줍 던 곳 ——
그 곳 이 차 마 꿈 — 엔 들 잊 힐 리 — 야

82

정재연

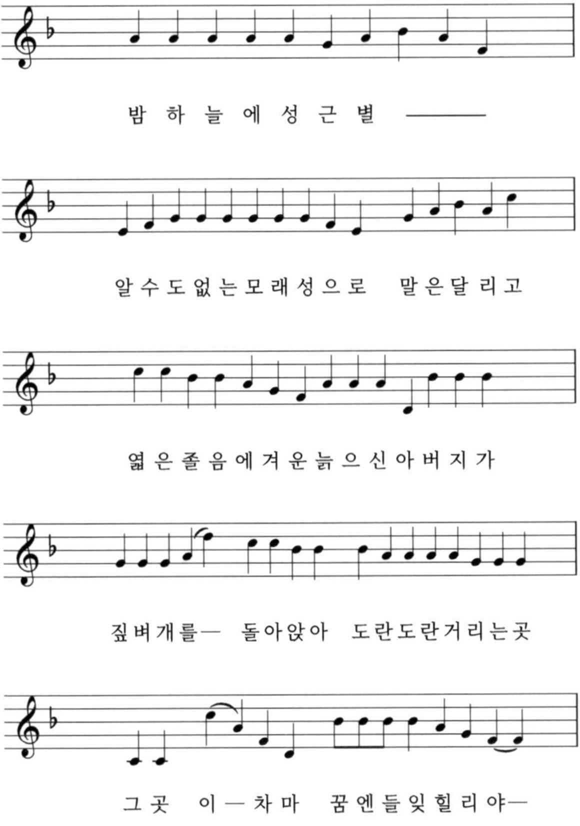
밤 하 늘 에 성 근 별 ———
알수도없는모래성으로 말은달리고
엷은졸음에겨운늙으신아버지가
짚벼개를— 돌아앉아 도란도란거리는곳
그곳 이—차마 꿈엔들잊힐리야—

2.

창밖은 어느새 깜깜해졌다.
아직 가사가 온전히 기억나지는 않지만, 더 이상 가사를 떠올리기엔 무리가 있다.
그 과정 자체로 의미가 있었다고 서둘러 결론을 짓는다.

이제 뭐하지?

사실 이곳에 온 목적은 딱히 없다.
독방 체험을 기대하기보다는, 남편이 추종하는 '고귀한 침묵의 명상'을 해볼 기회가 될 거라 생각했다.
그는 이 시설의 다른 방에 머무르고 있다. 이왕 온 김에 남편과 추억 하나 만들자 싶었다.

남편은 명상을 하기 시작하면서 여름마다 명상센터에 간다.
거기만 다녀오면 완전 다른 사람이 되는 것 같다.
일단 마음가짐이 긍정적으로 변하고 절제력이 높아진다.
특히 잘 참지 못하던 식욕을 억제하며 몸도 가벼워진다.
그러다 보니 삶에 대한 만족도가 높아지고 마음의 여유를 즐기게 된 듯하다.
그러나 그것도 유효기간이 있다.
스스로 몸과 마음이 산만해지는 듯싶으면 또 다시 명상에 돌입한다.
그러면 다시 충만한 상태가 된다.
남편 말로는 명상의 목적이 생각하지 않기 위해서란다.

그런데 정말 생각하지 않고 견딜 수 있을까?
나는 그게 제일 궁금했다.
그래서 이 방에서 생각하지 않는 상태를 경험할 것이라는 약간의 기대가 있었다.

그런데 여기서 나는 틈만 나면 자꾸 뭔가 하려고 애쓴다.
들어와서도 끊임없이 뭔가를 생각한다.
쉴 새 없이 창밖을 응시한다.
밖에서 소리가 들려온다.
곧 비가 내릴 듯한 신호가 들린다.
빗방울이 전선을 타고 흐르는 소리가 들린다.
왜가리가 나뭇가지에 앉아 털을 고르는 모습이 보인다.
안개가 하늘과 산을 가로지르는 장면이 지나간다.
간사님이 조용히 밥을 나르는 발자국 소리가 들린다.
동시에 괘종 시계가 고요함을 깨운다.

아, 이 모든 걸 경험하고 나면 노랫말이 또렷하게 되살아나려나.
그나저나 정지용의 고향은 어디였을까?
또 생각이란 걸 한다. 아무것도 하지 않는 게 진짜 어렵다.

어쩌면 창작 과정은 아무에게도 공개할 의무가 없고, 보여줄 필요도 없다는 전제로부터 시작되는 게 아닐까.

러셀 메이슨

여느 여름이 그렇듯, 밖에는 비가 계속해서 내린다. 나는 작은 방 안에 갇혀 있다. 하지만 나는 그다지 걱정하지 않는다. 한동안 나는 번갈아가며 가만히 앉아있어 보기도, 또 누워있어 보기도 해본다. 내부와 외부의 구별이 흐려질 때까지 내 몸 안팎 공간의 고요함과 침묵을 곱씹는다. 나는 반쯤 뜬 눈으로 내 앞에 있는, 나무가 울창한 숲을 응시한다. 그 공허한 장면에 초점을 맞추고 기다린다. 나의 초점이 그 순간에 맞춰지면, 맑은 빛이 나에게로 쏟아져 들어온다.

내가 보는 모든 것이 희미해져도 나는 편안하게 가만히 있다. 내 몸의 형상도 물에 비친 것처럼 옅어지며 깜박거린다. 이제 정신이 고요해졌으니, 주변 의식이 두드러지게 중요해진다. 나의 존재는 직감적으로 나 자신을 치유하기 시작한다. 정신적인 활동이 없는 상태에서는 완전한 존재와 안도감만이 존재한다. 그러다 하나의 생각이 꼬리에 꼬리를 물기 시작하며 이 행복의 바다에서 나를 끌어내 버린다. 지금 한 가지 나를 붙잡는 것이 있는데, 바로 이곳에 지내는 대가로 부탁을 받은 글쓰기이다.

머릿속에 단어가 맴돈다. 나는 글쓰기를 시작하기로 한다. *먼저 계약 조건을 이행하고, 정신의 소음을 배출한 다음 긴장을 풀고 명상에 집중하세요.* 방 안의 책상은 굉장히 낮고 불편해서 나의 무릎이나 팔꿈치가 이 불편함을 얼마나 견딜 수 있을지 확실하지 않다. 아마 나의 한국인 아내, 그리고 이 시설에 머무는 다른 사람들은 이러한 불편함에 개의치 않을 수도 있으리라 생각한다. 여기에선 인터넷 연결이 되지 않기 때문에, 나는 펜으로 종이에 글을 쓰고 있다. 학생일 때 부지런히 연마하여 능숙했던 글쓰기는 여러 해가 지나 이제는 어

찌지 부자연스럽다. 뇌 회로가 가소성을 역행하듯 나는 겨우 글자에 비슷한 모양을 형성할 수 있었다. 글쓰기는 나의 성적 역사의 기승전결을 따랐는데, 그것은 마치 끊임없는 흐름이 간헐적인 흘러내림으로 바뀌는 것과도 같았다.

미루기의 달콤한 위험을 인지하고 있기에, 나는 망설이지 않고 글을 쓰기 시작한다.

"명상하는 것과 백지 위에 글을 쓰는 것의 공통점은 두 행위 모두 우리가 내면을 직면할 수밖에 없는 상황에 놓이도록 한다는 점입니다. 명상 중에 떠오르는 단어처럼, 이 페이지에 글을 쓰면서 제게 떠오르는 단어들은 바로 이 순간 저의 생각 이외에 그 아무것도 될 수 없습니다."

'썩 나쁘지 않은데.' 하지만 이것들은 당신의 생각이 아니다. 당신은 단지 익숙한 사회적 담론에 따라 생각을 내면화했을 뿐이다. 나는 개의치 않고 계속한다.

"그러면 창문에 보이는 풀과 푸른 나무, 창백한 하늘은 어떻습니까? 분명히 그것은 제 마음속에 있는 생각이 아닙니다. 그것은 제 몸 밖의 시간과 공간에서 특정한 물리적 장소를 차지하고 있는 실제 세계의 물체입니다. 그런 물체는 결코 제 내면의 생각이라 할 수 없습니다. 아니면 이것은 단지 아직 검토되지 않은 가정일 뿐일까요?"

"하지만 사실 외부로부터 온전히 독립적인 관점은 결코 있을 수 없습니다. 나무, 내리쬐는 새하얀 빛, 그리고 우둔한 돌은 제 내면의 감각된 인식 혹은 매개 이미지입니다. 그 어떤 인간도 세상을 본 적도, 볼 수도 없었습니다. 우리는 모두 단지 내면의 내용을 들여다보고 이 혼란 속에서 '세계'라고 불리는 개념 혹은 그 집합체에 관해 겨우 말하거나 써 본 적이 있을

RUSSELL MASON

뿐입니다. 이러한 사실이 명백한데도, 그 누구도 그에 대해 깊이 생각하는 것 같지 않습니다. 대부분의 사람은 비록 그러한 세계가 결코 실재하지도 않았고 또 증명될 수도 없지만, 그들 자신의 인식 세계가 육체 바깥에서 일어나는 실제 경험의 틀림없는 대상이라는 믿음을 고집합니다. 하지만 이러한 믿음은 단지 수반하는 논의를 의미 있게 하는 가정일 뿐입니다. 그렇더라도 이쯤에서 잠시 멈춰서 이 가정에 대해 우리가 무엇을 할 수 있을지 생각해봅시다."

"우리가 깨어 있는 삶을 고려해보면, 우리는 *몸이거나 몸 '안'에 있는 것처럼* 보이고, 그 몸은 그것 밖의 세계를 경험하게 됩니다. 기본적으로 몸과 그 안의 것, 그리고 그 밖에 있는 세계나 우주라는 두 점이 있는 것 같습니다. 그런데 우리가 이미 잘못된 방향을 선택한 걸까요? 불필요하게 두 번째 사실을 추가했을까요? 우리의 경험에 근거하여 제 실제는 단지 하나의 몸 또는 몸 '안'에 있는 것일 뿐 동시에 몸 바깥에 늘 존재하는 공간이 아니라는 걸 입증하는, 합리적 의심을 넘는 근거나 증거가 있을까요? 물론 대부분은 우리가 말하는 *내면*의 생각, 느낌, 감각 그리고 감정에 대한 직접적인 경험을 가지고 있습니다. 이것이 말하는 습관과 내면의 개념에 대한 믿음보다 더욱 실질적인 것으로 드러날까요? 내면성과 외면성에 대한 개념이 없다면, 감각과 감정은 여전히 경험됩니다. 단순히 신체의 피부라는 경계에서 멈추지 않고 더 확장된 연속체에 대한 인식을 경험할 수 있습니다. 하지만 우리는 마치 미개봉한 수프 통 같습니다. 우리는 정형화된 상징에 무척이나 익숙해져 있습니다. 그래서 문화적으로 특정한 기호학을 통해 세상을 안팎으로 정의하고, 그에 따른 삶을 사는 데 능숙합니

다. 왜냐하면 우리는 마치 드넓은 바다가 우리의 제어된 피부 안에 응축되어 있다고 생각하며 서투르게 정의 내리기를 좋아하기 때문입니다."

이 문장을 마무리 지으며 내 생각을 분석하는 행동 자체가 나의 존재에 대한 지각을 감소시킨다는 것을 깨닫게 된다. 마치 내가 표현하고 싶은 의식의 방식을 경험할 수 없게 만드는 것처럼 말이다.

"몸과 몸 밖의 공간은 우리의 깨어 있는 삶에서 늘 존재하는 사실인데, 우리는 어떻게 우리가 두 가지가 아니라 단지 하나라는 것을 *알* 수 있습니까? 더 나아가 가장 근본적인 차원에서, 어떻게 여러분이 심지어 이 두 가지 중 하나라는 것을 알 수 있습니까? 우리 모두에게 육체와 우주는 지각의 대상으로, 혹은 우리 안에 있는 것으로 보입니다. 개체는 인식의 대상으로 나타날 수 있습니까? 당신은 시간과 함께 사라지는 모든 형태, 물체 그리고 경험을 인지하고, 행위자 또는 과정 자체가 될 수 있습니까? 당신이 만약 본인에게 정말로 솔직하다면 모른다고 인정할 것입니다. 이 사실을 인정하며 절망이 찾아올 때, 또 알려고 하는 모든 노력을 포기할 때, 그리고 당신이 너무나 깊이 사랑에 빠진 거짓된 자아의 모든 극본을 포기할 때 — 바로 그렇게 모른다는 것을 인정할 때 비로소 더 많은 것을 알 준비가 됩니다. 여태껏 당신은 과장된 자신만의 환상에서 살고 있었습니다. 당신은 자신이 세상을 온전히 이해하는 특별한 존재라는 꿈을 꾸며, 그 환상을 유지하기 위해 가능한 모든 노력을 하고 있었습니다."

"우리 대부분이 사는 이 감옥은 어떤 이유로 생겨나는 것일까요? 부분적으로는, 별개의 대상에 대한 믿음에서 비롯됩

니다. 생각, 감각, 고통, 나무, 심지어 단어 같은 특정 '내부' 또는 '외부' 대상에 주의를 집중시킴으로써, 우리는 그 대상이 실제로 맥락과 의미를 부여하는 우주의 나머지 부분과 분리되어 있음을 알게 됩니다. 이것은 사소한 문제가 아닙니다. 그 대상의 연속적인 전환 상태에서 살아가는 것이 우리가 꽤나 관심을 기울이는 부분이기 때문입니다. 특정한 대상, 목표, 환상, 사랑의 대상, 심지어 환상적 사랑의 대상에 대한 욕망은 우리를 고립의 세계에서 계속 부유하게 합니다. 이러한 의미에서 감옥은 우리의 욕망, 두려움과 추측 그리고 세상을 이해하려 하는 노력과 투쟁으로 구성되어 있습니다. 쾌락과 지식을 추구하는 본성을 가진 우리는 객체가 우리 외부에 존재하고 그러한 대상에 일시적으로 매료되며, 그것에 대한 갈망이 잠시 중단될 때 욕망이 충족됐다고 오해합니다. 그 대상이 결코 우리의 본질적 욕구를 충족시켜 주지 못한다는 것을 반복된 경험을 통해 배우지만, 우리는 쉬이 그것을 이해하지 못합니다. 사실 우리가 추구하는 각각의 대상은 그 대상에 대한 열망을 포기해야만 얻을 수 있는 것으로서, 고요함에 대한 진정한 욕망으로 가장한 2차적 욕망입니다. 즉, 우리가 취하는 모든 행동은 마지막 행동이 될 것이라는 희망으로 이루어집니다. 그러나 우리는 이 모든 거짓된 대체물에서 이를 찾는 것을 포기하면 진정한 본성을 경험할 수 있습니다."

이곳에 온 지 두 시간이 채 안 되었을 때, 오랫동안 나를 괴롭히던 서양 중심적 사고에 대한 문제를 바로 이 부분에서 거의 해결했다. 나중에 이에 대해 더 자세하게 말하겠다. 난 마치 순수한 자각의 호수에 잠겨 시간을 보내는 듯한 보상을 확실히 받았다.

온전히 가만히 누워 내 몸에 집중한다. 그러나 나는 안도할 수도 긴장을 완전히 풀 수도 없다. 내 내면에 떠오르는 글에 대해 곰곰이 생각한다.

어두워지는 하늘을 바라보며 문득 생각한다. *나는 이 방에서 나갈 수 없다.* 이 사실에 대해 꼭 당황하고 있는 것은 아니지만, 이는 찌릿한 전율을 불러일으킨다. 창문을 열고 신선한 공기를 마신다. *당신은 이 방에 지금부터 열다섯 시간을 더 있어야 합니다.* 나는 센터에서 일하는 자원봉사자가 밖에서 걸어 다니는 것을 지켜본다. 비록 그들처럼 비를 맞고 싶은 마음은 없지만, 나는 그들의 자유를 본능적으로 증오한다.

이 덧없는 생각의 연속에서 한동안 앉아 있다가 시간이 얼마나 느리게 흘러가고 있는지 알게 된다. 바깥의 시계가 정시를 알릴 때, 나는 너무 피곤해서 글을 쓰거나 명상을 할 수도 없을 정도로 무기력해진다.

뜻밖에도 나는 분노에 찬 비명을 지르고, 방문을 덜컹 두드리고 싶은 욕망으로 가득 차 있다. 내 생각은 하향 곡선에 빠져 있다. 감옥에 있는 사람들이 자주 느끼는 분노, 지루함, 무의미함을 잠시나마 엿볼 수 있었다. 자유를 박탈하는 것 자체가 벌이라는 명백한 통찰력을 얻을 만할 정도로 말이다.

가능한 한 속히 잠들고 싶어 불을 끈다. 얼른 오늘 하루를 마무리 짓고 싶다. 하지만 어둠 속에 누워 있으니, 실제 감옥에서 자는 것이 얼마나 어려울까 하는 생각이 꼬리에 꼬리를 문다. 과민한 정신이 만들어내는 가상의 위협은 그 아무리 좋을 때라도 불쾌하기 마련이다. 그렇다면 수용된 사람들이 실제로 맞닥뜨리는 위협은 얼마나 더 끔찍할까? 나는 속히 잠에 들길 바라지만, 한편으론 깨어 있다. 쉴 새 없는 생각

은 어설픈 애송이 도둑마냥 내가 자연스레 잠들기 전까지 비틀거리며 돌아다닌다.

나는 놀라울 정도로 개운한 아침을 맞이한다. 아침에 눈을 뜨니 전날 밤보다 훨씬 더 가뿐하다. 자명종 소리는 마치 아기의 장난감 음악상자처럼 꽤 감미롭기도 하다. 계속되는 소리에 자명종 시계를 찾지만, 그 어디에서도 찾을 수 없다. 감미로운 음악은 이내 성가신 음악이 된다. 나는 여느 아침처럼 성급히 탁자 위 벽에 있는 버튼이나 스위치를 찾으려 한다. *내 허락 없이 찾아온 이 우스꽝스러운 음악 때문에 미칠 것 같다.*

몇 분 후, 이윽고 자명종 소리가 멈추고 108배를 알리는 녹음 음성이 나온다. 한국에서 흔히 볼 수 있는 이 불교 풍습은 행복공장의 대표가 강력하게 추천한 것이었다. 목소리의 안내에 따라 나는 어색하고 서투른 자세로 고개를 숙이지만, 그와 반대로 내 마음은 원망과 분노로 가득하다. 나는 진심으로 감사하는 태도를 가질 때까지 108배를 계속할 수 없다고 결심한다. 명상 자세로 앉아 내 삶을 크게 향상시켜준 영적 스승들의 이미지를 떠올린다. 먼저 석가모니, 노자, 파드마삼바, 틸로파, 아디 샹카라, 마이스터 에크하르트에게 감사의 인사를 전한다. 이내 내 몸은 심장 중앙에서 흐르는 온화한 에너지의 파도로 가득 차기 시작한다. 텐진 왕걀 린포체, S.N. 고엔카, 사야 기 우 바킨, 레디 사야도에게 감사의 마음을 전할 때에는 온화한 에너지의 물결이 내 몸의 빈자리를 채우고 몸 밖의 자리와 합쳐진다. 그리고 코로나로 인해 담마 코리아 명상 센터가 문을 닫기 전까지 함께했던 명상 수련회 선생님과 동료가 생각난다. 세계에서 손꼽히는 영적인 전통으로부터 영감 받은 강연을 온라인으로 제공해준 호주의 여승 사마

네리 자야사도 떠오른다. 나는 그렇게 내 삶에서 유영하는 사람들에게 감사함을 전하기로 한다. 나의 아내와 영국, 한국의 가족, 그리고 내 친구와 멘토들에게.

감사함을 전하는 행위의 중요성에 대해 익히 알고 있고, 심지어 실천하기 위해 노력하기도 했지만 나는 우리 대부분이 주로 하는 관례대로만 해왔다. 나에게 베푼 친절을 잊지 않으며 그것에 답례하는 정도로 말이다. 하지만 이것은 껍데기에 불과하다. 그동안 나는 마음에서 진정으로 우러나오는 감사의 마음을 놓치고 있었다는 것을 알게 되었다. 이 깨달음 덕에 여태껏 나를 도와준 분들에 대한 깊은 감사의 물결이 내 무의식 깊은 곳에서 솟아오른다. 이러한 감정은 벅차오르기도, 또 금세 차분해지기도 한다. 이 감사의 마음이 나를 오랫동안 휘저었던 불안을 휩쓸어 내버리면서, 나는 모든 생명의 상호연계성에 대해 더욱 선명하게 알게 된다.

108배 기록이 마무리될 때, 나는 생경한 고요함 속에서 기본적인 통찰이 이렇게나 선명하다는 것에 감명을 받았다. 이 글쓰기의 과정은 나를 분석적인 사고방식으로 되돌아가게 했다. 최대한의 노력에도 불구하고 나는 정신 활동의 감옥으로 떨어졌는데, 그 안에서 분리된 몸이 된 경험은 아주 현실적이었다. 이런 정신 상태에서 의식의 통일성을 깨닫는 건 불가능하다. 술에 취한 사람이 단순히 상상만으로 술에서 깨어나려는 것처럼 말이다.

이런 생각들이 피어오르면서, 시간과 공간의 사이는 확장되고 현실의 순차적 본질은 다시 사라진다. 몇 시간이 지나 집에서 노트북으로 글을 끝맺고 있는 지금, 마지막으로 생각이 나는 건 내가 말하고 싶은 것 중 그 어떤 것도 말로 표현될

수 없다는 사실이 이 글의 도입부가 되어야 한다는 것이다. 사실 이는 내가 몇 년 전 작가가 되고 싶다는 환상을 버린 이유이기도 하다. 행복공장에 머무르는 것은 과거의 내 모습을 되살릴 수 있는 기회였을 뿐만 아니라, 차마 솔직하게 말할 수 없어 두 번 다시 말하지 않기로 한 것들을 표현해 볼 수 있는 편리한 핑계이기도 했다. 비 오는 울창한 숲에 둘러싸인 그 작은 방에 대한 기억이 차츰 옅어져 간다. 그리고 확신하건대, 나는 이 모든 것에 감사하다.

여인영

「유기체 안으로 오르가즘 구부리기」

표면은 평평하다

평평한 ***구멍(hole)***[1]의 끝이 보이기 시작한다. 그 구멍은 한 개의 점에서 정사각형과 원 사이의 어떤 모양으로 픽셀화된다. 위에 일곱 개의 구멍이 돌출하기 시작한다. 그리고 천천히 3차원적으로 보이기 시작한다. 한 부분이 회전한다. 두 개의 구멍이 서로의 주위를 돌고 돈다. 세 부분이 서로를 회전한다. 네 개의 점이 한 쌍으로 회전하며 다른 점들과 교체하여 서로의 주위를 돌고 돈다. 둘, 셋으로 이루어진 한 쌍의 부분들이 서로의 주위를 돌고 돈다. 여섯이 함께 모여 세 개의 쌍으로 나뉘어 회전한다. 일곱 개의 부분들은 그들 안에서 회전하고 또 다른 이들 주위를 돌고 돈다. 그 회전이 다시 시작한다. 돌고 도는 한 개의 중심축은 새로 회전을 시작할 때마다 그 과정과 경로가 한 눈금씩 이동한다.

나는 분명 어느 한 개의 지점을 기준으로 회전하는 것 같다. 그럼 이곳은 시공간의 어디쯤일까? 구멍? ***부분(parts)***[2]? 전체? 세로로 그 시작점에서 끝의 점까지와 가로로 그 시작점에서 끝의 점까지의 길이는 동일하게 측정된다. 그 구멍의 전체 개수를 세어보면 열두 개의 부분적인 구멍인데 즉 (1,1,0,0), (1,0,1,0), (1,0,0,1), (0,1,0,1), (0,0,1,1), (0,1,1,0)이 된다. 한 부분이 이탈한다. 숫자 '0' 한 개는 그 자리를 유지한다. 둘은 함께 작동하여 ***전체(whole)***[3], 즉 커다랗고 평평한 구멍이 될 때까지 구멍들 속으로 빠진다.

표면은 평평하다. 표면은 회전하고, 곡선을 이루며, 구부러지

고 또 접힌다. 표면은 3차원인 동시에 계속해서 평평해진다.

슈퍼 계란이 탄생한다.

1 : 하나는 네모난 상자로 가득 차 있고 하나는 곡선으로 가득 차 있다.

0 : 끝에서부터 시작하자.
1 : 당신의 끝? 아니면 나의 끝?
0 : 우리의 끝에서 시작하자.
1 : 우리의 최종 목표는 편리함이야.
0 : 그게 바로 시작이야.
1 : 그건 한 부분이지. 전체 구멍은 어때?
0 : 한 개의 상자에는 여섯 개의 면이 있는데 그럼 전체 구멍에는 몇 개의 면이 있나?
1 : 구멍에는 360도 곡선이 있어.
0 : 그 곡선을 얇게 베어내 그것으로 네모난 상자를 만들어 보자.

0 : 알겠다.
1 : 얇게 베어낸 곡선을 평평하게 펴봐.

1 : 나는 한 개의 면이 보인다.
0 : 나는 ***두 극단***[4]이 보인다.
1 : 나는 세 개의 면이 보인다.
0 : 나는 네 개의 면이 보인다.

1 : 나는 다섯 개의 면이 보인다.

0 : 나는 0 개의 면이 보여. 나는 곡선이 보인다.

1 : 네모난 상자의 여섯 개 면을 평평하게 펼치고, 구멍의 360도 곡선에 맞춰서 돌려봐.

0 : 그래, 그렇게 해보지. 그 안에는 무엇이 있어?

1 : 모든 것은 안에 있고 모든 것은 바깥에 있어.

0 : 표면은 ***투명***[5]이고, 반투명이며, 반-불투명이며, 불투명이다. 이것은 반영하며, 비추고, 소용돌이치며, 차별화하며, 연결하며, 차단하며, 흡수하며… '하고 있고' 하고 있다.

1 : 얼마나 깊어?

0 : 그것은 내부적으로, 외부적으로, 수평으로, 수직으로, 대각선으로 그리고 표면과 깊이에서 모든 방향으로 깊이를 가지고 있다.

1 : 우리는 어디서 만나?

0 : 나는 너를 만난다.

1 : 나는 너를 만난다.

0 : 우리는 만난다.

1 : 내가 만나고, 네가 만나고, 우리가 만나고, 그들이 우리를 만난다.

0 : 어디서?

1 : 하나는 네모난 상자로 가득 차 있고 하나는 곡선으로 가득 차 있다.

표면을 펼쳐 구멍 안 곡선에 맞추어 구부리기

곡선과 평면이 시야를 만들어준다. 내 눈동자의 구멍에서 곡선이 돌아 나를 향해 돌아온다. 스쳐 지나가는 불빛을 놓쳤나 확인한다. 그 어느 것도 그대로 머물지 않지만, 시간은 다시 흘러가기 시작한다. 가볍게 *두드리고(tap), 클릭(click)*하고, *넘기지(swipe)* 않으면 무슨 뜻인지 모르겠다. 그래서 다른 곳으로 시선을 돌린다. 함께 공유할 수 있는 녹음과 친구를 찾는다. 평평한 평면에 평평하게 몸을 펼친다. 얼굴의 표면이 360도 돌아가는데 측면으로도, 수직으로도 혹은 수평으로도 아닌, 기이하게 구부러진다. 나는 물 웅덩이에 흘러들어간다. 어쩐지 그 파란색이 무거워지면서 나를 다른 면으로 뒤집는다. 나는 위로 부유해 앉고, 곡선은 멈추기 시작한다. 몸은 움직임이 없는 구멍에 맞춰 평평해진다. 안쪽을 들여다보면 화려한 손톱들이 서로 만나기 위해 구부러진다. 서로를 만나기 어려워지면서, 그들은 서로가 서로의 주위를 돌고 돌며 끊임없이 우회한다. 이 경로와 형태가 새로운 ***패턴***[6]을 형성하면서 엄지 손가락이 쿵, 쿵, 쿵 두드리기 시작한다. 한 번의 두드림으로도 진동이 느껴진다. 이는 실수나 우연처럼 느껴지지만 아마도 나는 이 모든 것을 아주 의도적으로, 나의 ***욕망***[7]을 충족시키려는 평평한 목표를 향해 간 것 같다.

당신을 만질 수 없어, 나는 가장 친한 친구를 데려와 내가 만질 수 있는 가능한 모든 것을 만진다. 따뜻하지는 않지만 쉽고, 편리하기도 하고, 때로는 아주 화려하다. 얼굴이 움직이고, 흐르고, 내 얼굴 주위를 회전할 때, 나는 그저 얼굴의 표

면을 벗어 다른 얼굴을 마주한다. 얼굴을 마주하는 것과 얼굴을 벗기는 행위는 층위를 이루어 평평하고 넓은 곡선이 되고, 나는 그 위를 걸어 넘어간다. 나의 친밀감에는 한계가 없지만, 나는 구부려 질문한다.

2 : 목표는 편리함이다.
0 : 작은 구멍들이 보인다.
1 : 작은 구멍들? 어디에?

1 : 내 네모난 상자들 안에.

0 : 내게 ***정보(information)***[8]를 주면 질문을 찾아볼게.
1 : 목표는 구멍 안에 소변을 보고, 빨간 'x'들을 모으고, 상자를 두드러지게 하는 것이다. 당신은 구멍들이야.

1 : 상자 너머 있는 스타킹들은 'x'의 것인가?
0 : 내 생각에 그것은 노란색이야.
1 : 그것을 노랑으로 생각하면서 목표가 구멍에 소변을 보는 것이라면, 당신이 내 작은 구멍들을 사랑한다는 뜻인가?
0 : 그렇다 그리고 아니다.

1 : 시나리오 〈그렇다〉
0 : 구멍은 점이다.
1 : 가까이서 보면 평평한 검은색 점이다.
0 : 구멍이 증식하여 전체로 커진다.

1 : 나는 당신이 증식할 때가 좋아.
0 : 얼굴을 구멍에 넣어보라. 기분이 어떤가?
1 : 회전하고 있다.
0 : '0'과 '1'을 이끌고 따르는 숫자들 속에서 당신의 얼굴을 벗어봐.
2 : 목표는 편리함이다.

0 : 시나리오 〈아니다〉
1 : 구멍은 아무것도 아니다.
0 : 두 엄지손가락을 위한 두 개의 구멍들.
1 : 완벽하다.
2 : 목표는 편리함이다.

1 : 시나리오 〈영 '0'〉
0 : 구멍은 전체이고, 전체는 구멍의 부분이고 전체이며 다시 구멍이다.
1 : '0'은 시작과 끝을 표시한다.
0 : 이는 무한하다.
2 : 목표는 편리함이다.

2 : 목표는 편리함이다.

유기체 속의 오르가즘

숨이 차서 죽는 느낌의 두려움 그리고 내 자신 안의 인내의 끝점에 다다른 이 고문의 무한 반복, 그것은 죽음, 끝이 없는 죽음처럼 느껴진다. 상상할 수 있는가? 끝이 없는 죽음을? 숨을 헐떡이는 것이 이토록 생기 있게 느껴진 적이 없다.

열은 욕망과 즐거움의 공간을 충족시켜준다. 어떤 한 개의 부분은 전체가 아닌 구멍에 속하기에, 그 뜨거운 욕망은 모든 부분을 채운다. 벽, 창문, 그리고 빛으로부터 ***소외***[9]되고 지쳐 '나는 잠이 든다.' 실재는 거짓보다 더 실재 같으며, 실재보다 더 거짓 같다. 단 한 번의 신체적 접촉도 없이, 전체의 구멍이, 그 이상의 감각을 느낀다. '오(Oh)'라는 감탄사, 알파벳 오 'O'와 숫자 영 '0'은 돌고 또 돈다. 빙글빙글 돈다. 그들은 360도 차원에서 돌고 돌며 '공(空)'으로 돌아간다. 이곳에서 모든 것이 시작하고 끝나며, 부분 그리고 구멍들과 함께 다시금 '전체'가 된다.

0 : 나는 ***순환 고리(loop)***[10]를 돌고있다.
1 : 나는 발기한다. 나는 관통한다. 나는 식민화한다. 이 고리는 내 것이다. 나의 승리이다.
0 : 나는 소용돌이친다. 나는 공유한다. 나는 비워낸다.
1 : 나는 이해할 수 없다. 말이 되지 않는다.
0 : 너는 유일무이한 기표가 아니다.
1 : 내가 바로 정답이다.
0 : 나는 질문이 많다. 다음 질문은 무엇인가? 부분, 구멍에

서 전체까지, ***'0'과 '1'(zeros and ones)***[11]을 이끌고 따르는 숫자들 속에서.

1 : 창문이 없는 거울이 보인다. 그리고 그것은 다른 이에게 화려한 것들로 가득 찬 그의 권력을 반사한다.

0 : 내 안의 거울은 끈적이면서도 부드럽고, 공허하고 반투명하면서도 가득 차 있으며, 반영하고, 보답하고, 또 순환한다.

1 : 나는 무엇을 얻는가?

0 : 이것은 순환 고리이다. 그 누구도 무엇을 얻지 못하고 또한 모든 사람이 무언가를 얻는다. 이는 곧 나선형의 순환이다.

1 : 순환 고리이므로, 새로운 고리로 시작한다. 나는 알파벳 오 'o'와 숫자 영 '0'을 원한다.

0 : 새로운 나선형 고리에서는 알파벳 'o'는 없지만 '0'과 '1'의 복합 숫자들이 존재한다.

0 : 이것은 개방형 나선형이다.

1 : 나는 소문자 알파벳 'o'를 원한다.

0 : 나는 대문자 알파벳 'O'를 원한다.

1 : 나는 숫자 영 '0'을 원한다.

0 : 나는 구멍을 원한다.

1 : 방을 닫아라.

0 : 방을 열어라.

1 : 나는 순환 고리를 돌고 있다.

나선형 순환의 시뮬라시옹[12]

■ *대본*

0 : ***실재***[13]란 무엇인가?
1 : 세 가지로 설명하자면,

1 : 주체, 매개체, 객체,
0 : ***전체(whole)***[14], 부분, 구멍,
1 : 관찰자, 번역자, 수신자,
0 : 나는 매혹된다.
1 : 얼굴은 휘어지고,
0 : 평평해지고,
1 : 이것은 하나의 얼굴이며,
0 : 이것은 영 '0'인 동시에 많은 얼굴이자, 하나의 얼굴로 베어낸 층위이고,
1 : 이것은 하나의 정답이며,
0 : 이것은 영 '0'인 동시에 많은 질문이자, 하나의 정답으로 베어낸 대답들이고,
1 : 나는 혼란스럽고,
0 : 나는 궁금하다.

0 : 나선형을 돌고 돌아와, 실재란 무엇인가?
1 : ***파생실재(hyperreality)***[15]를 상상해보라,
0 : 영('0')과 일('1')들,

1 : 표면들,
0 : 통일되기 위해 차별화하고,
1 : 얼굴의 차이가 표면으로 드러나면서 ***조직화(organize)***[16]되고,
0 : 평평함은 회전하며 휘어지고,
1 : 방을 닫으면,
0 : 평평해지고,
1 : 방을 열면,
0 : 휘어지고,
1 : 일 '1'들과 영 '0'들,
0 : 나선형 고리로 돌아와, 실재란 무엇인가?
1 : 구멍(HOLE), 전체(WHOLE), 오르가즘(ORGASM), 그리고 ***유기체(ORGANISM)***[17]의 대문자 오 'O',
0 : 꺼내고,
1 : 사라지기 위해 등장하고,
0 : 얼굴은 ***통일(unification)***[18] 속에서 휘어지면서 평평해지고, 평평해지면서 휘어지고,
1 : 욕망하고,

1 : 욕망을 향해 다시금 접히고,
0 : 나선형으로 돌아가,

1. "But this fault, this deficiency, this '***hole***,' inevitably affords woman too few figurations, images, or representations by which to represent herself. It is not that she lacks some 'master signifier' or that none is imposed upon her, but rather that access to a signifying economy, to the coining of signifiers, is difficult or even impossible for her because she remains an outsider, herself (a) subject to their norms." Luce Irigaray, *Speculum of the Other Woman* (1974; Ithaca: Cornell University Press, 1985), 71. *필자 주: 강조를 위해 볼드 및 이탤릭으로 임의 표기하였으며, 참고문헌의 번역본이 국내에 출판되지 않아 영문 본문을 유지하였다.

2. "사이보그의 경계 침범의 이면에는 해러웨이가 말하는 닿아서는 안되는 ***부분들***의 '쾌락적일 만큼 밀접한 짝짓기'가 존재한다. 사이보그는 에로틱한 침범을 강력하고 새로운 융합과 뒤섞기 때문에 종종 계급, 민족, 문화적 차이를 나타내 왔던 신체적 경계 논쟁의 무대가 된다." 캐서린 헤일즈, 『우리는 어떻게 포스트휴먼이 되었는가』, 허진 역(파주: 열린책들, 2013), 162. *필자 주: 강조를 위해 볼드 및 이탤릭으로 임의 표기하였다.

"Recursion is the movement that tirelessly integrates contingency into its own functioning to realize its telos. In so doing it generates an impenetrable complexity in the course of time. Organisms exhibit a complexity of relations between ***parts*** and whole inside the body and with its environment (e.g., structural coupling) in its functioning." Yuk Hui, *Recursivity and Contingency* (London: Rowman & Littlefield, 2019), 15. *필자 주: 강조를 위해 볼드 및 이탤릭으로 임의 표기하였으며, 참고문헌의 번역본이 국내에 출판되지 않아 영문 본문을 유지하였다.

3. "She is 'not-all,' 'not-***whole***,' 'not-one,' and whatever she knows can only be described as 'not-knowledge.' […] She has no place like home, nothing of her own, 'other than the place of the Other which,' writes Lacan, 'I designate with a capital O.'" Sadie Plant, *Zeros and Ones: Digital Women and the New Technoculture* (New York: Doubleday, 1997), 35. *필자 주: 강조를 위해 볼드 및 이탤릭으로 임의 표기하였으며, 참고문헌의 번역본이 국내에 출판되지 않아 영문 본문

을 유지하였다.

4. "곡선형 거울의 ***두 극단***들처럼 시스템과 그의 대체적인 극의 결합, 차후로 자성을 띠고 순환적이며 우파에서 좌파로 되돌아가는 정치적 공간의 '악순환적인' 휨, 전환의 고약한 천재인 뒤틀림으로서 ***모든*** 시스템, 즉 자본의 무한은 자기자신의 무한? 표면 위로 되돌아와 겹쳐진다. 욕망과 무의식적 성적 욕망의 공간도 마찬가지 아닌가? 욕망과 가치의 결합, 욕망과 자본의 결합." 장 보드리야르, 『시뮬라시옹』, 하태환 역(서울: 민음사, 2001), 50–52. *필자 주: 강조를 위해 볼드 및 이탤릭으로 임의 표기하였다.

5. "'진실' 경험 속에서는 비밀이나 변태의 문제가 아니라, 실재의 전율 혹은 파생실재의 미학이라는 문제가 있다. 현기증 나고 속은 듯한 정확성의 전율, 거리가 떨어지면서 동시에 확대되는 전율, 축척이 뒤틀린 전율, 과도한 ***투명***성의 전율이다." Ibid., 66–67. *필자 주: 강조를 위해 볼드 및 이탤릭으로 임의 표기하였다.

6. "이러한 전환이 가장 명확하게 드러난 텍스트를 정보 내러티브라고 부른다. [...] 우리는 어떤 시대에든 ***패턴***에 초점을 맞출 수 있지만, 정보 내러티브 ***패턴***의 특징은 임의성에 깊이 침투당해 있으며 은연중에 물질성에 도전한다는 점이다. ***패턴***은 현존을 압도하고, 따라서 정신이나 의식이 아니라 오직 정보에만 의존하는 탈물질성이 구성된다." 헤일즈, 80. *필자 주: 강조를 위해 볼드 및 이탤릭으로 임의 표기하였다.

"임의성은 ***패턴***에 구멍을 뚫어 배경의 화이트 노이즈가 쏟아져 들어오게 만든다." Ibid., 439. *필자 주: 강조를 위해 볼드 및 이탤릭으로 임의 표기하였다.

"오른쪽 부재와 ***패턴***의 상호작용은 장 보드리야르를 따라 극실재라고 부를 수 있다." Ibid., 441. *필자 주: 강조를 위해 볼드 및 이탤릭으로 임의 표기하였다.

7. "'정신분석' 은 심지어 ***욕망***에 결핍이라는 부정적 법칙을, 쾌락이라는 외적 규칙을, 환상이라는 초월적 이상을 새겨 넣는 새로운 수단을 발견했다." 질 들뢰즈, 펠릭스 가타리, 『천 개의 고원』, 김재인 역(서울: 새물결, 2001), 297. *필자 주: 강조를 위해 볼드 및 이탤릭으로 임의 표기하였다.

"CsO(기관이 없는 몸체)가 고른판 또는 ***욕망***의 내재성의 장이어서만은 아니다. 설령 CsO가 조잡한 탈지층화의 공허함에 빠지거나 암적인 지층의 증식에 빠지더라도 그것은 여전히 ***욕망***이다. ***욕망***은 자신의 소멸을 욕망하거나 소멸할 수 있는 역량을 갖는 자가 되기를 욕망하는 단계까지 가기도 한다. 돈의 ***욕망***, 군대의 ***욕망***, 경찰과 국가의 ***욕망***, 파시스트-***욕망***, 파시즘조차도 ***욕망***인 것이다." Ibid., 316. *필자 주: 강조를 위해 볼드 및 이탤릭으로 임의 표기하였다.

"그러나 여성은 단순히 자신의 생산품으로부터 소외될 뿐 아니라 깊은 의미에서 주체로, 혹은 잠재적 주체로도 존재하지 않는다. 왜냐하면 여성은 여자로서의 자신의 존재를 성적 전용에 빚지고 있기 때문이다. 다른 사람의 ***욕망***에 의해 구성된다는 것은 근로자가 자신의 생산품으로부터 폭력적으로 분리되면서 소외당하는 것과 동일하지 않다." 도나 해러웨이, 『유인원, 사이보그, 그리고 여자: 자연의 재발명』, 민경숙 역(서울: 동문선, 2002), 286. *필자 주: 강조를 위해 볼드 및 이탤릭으로 임의 표기하였다.

8. "***Information***, which is neither energy nor matter, demands a new place in ontology and reconstitutes the relations between other categories, as well as the foundations of knowledge, just as Bateson and Simondon did by bringing information together with recursion. It reacts against the tendency of separating active form from inert matter in classical metaphysics [...]." Hui, 148. *필자 주: 강조를 위해 볼드 및 이탤릭으로 임의 표기하였으며, 참고문헌의 번역본이 국내에 출판되지 않아 영문 본문을 유지하였다.

9. "칼 프리드먼은 라캉, 들뢰즈, 가타리 등 여러 학자들이 이론화했듯이 정신분열증을 가진 주체는 ***소외***된 '나'와 ***소외***시키는 '내가 아닌 것' 사이의 상호 작용을 통해서 발전한다고 지적한다." 헤일즈, 300. *필자 주: 강조를 위해 볼드 및 이탤릭으로 임의 표기하였다.

10. "The Chthulucene does not close in on itself; it does not round off; its contact zones are ubiquitous and continuously spin out ***loopy*** tendrils. Spider is a much better future for sympoiesis than any inadequately leggy vertebrate of whatever pantheon. Tentacularity is symchthonic, wound with abyssal and dreadful graspings,

frayings, and weavings, passing relays again and again, in the generative recursions that make up living and dying." Donna J. Haraway, *Staying with the Trouble* (Durham: Duke University Press, 2016), 33. *필자 주: 강조를 위해 볼드 및 이탤릭으로 임의 표기하였으며, 참고문헌의 번역본이 국내에 출판되지 않아 영문 본문을 유지하였다.

11. "[...] the ***zeros and ones*** of machine code do far more than hark back to the binaries their logical symbols represent. [...] In both electronic systems and the punched cards of weaving machines, a hole is one, and a blank is zero, in which case there are two missing elements, if missing is where either can be said to go. No longer a world of ones and not-ones, or something and nothing, thing and gap, but rather not-holes and holes, not-nothing and nothing, gap and not-gap." Plant, 56–57. *필자 주: 강조를 위해 볼드 및 이탤릭으로 임의 표기하였으며, 참고문헌의 번역본이 국내에 출판되지 않아 영문 본문을 유지하였다.

"우리가 비생물 매체–예를 들면 컴퓨터 디스크–에서 ***1과 0***의 형상을 파악할 수 있다면 육체라는 쓸데없는 살덩이가 왜 필요하겠는가?" 헤일즈, 41. *필자 주: 강조를 위해 볼드 및 이탤릭으로 임의 표기하였다.

12. "반면에 ***시뮬라시옹***은 '참'과 '거짓', '실재'와 '상상세계' 사이의 다름 자체를 위협한다." 보드리야르, 19. *필자 주: 강조를 위해 볼드 및 이탤릭으로 임의 표기하였다.

"딕크의 단편들은 '단번에 근원도 없고, 내재적이며, 과거도 없고 미래도 없는 ***시뮬라시옹*** 속에, (정신적, 시간적, 공간적, 기호적인) 모든 상관요소들의 부유 속에 있게 된다. 평행한 세계, 이중적인 세계, 혹은 가능한 세계의 문제도 아니다. 그것은 가능한, 불가능한, 실제의 비현실의 세계가 아니라 ***시뮬라시옹***의 세계이다." Ibid., 203. *필자 주: 강조를 위해 볼드 및 이탤릭으로 임의 표기하였다.

13. "시뮬라시옹의 과정을 실질적으로 격리시키기가 불가능하다면 우리를 둘러싸고 있는 ***실재***를 무기력하게 만드는 힘에 의해서 그 반대도 또한 진실이다 (그리고 이러한 회귀성조차도 권력을 시뮬라시옹으로 무력하게 하는

장치에 속한다). 즉 차후로는 ***실재***의 과정을 분리하거나, 실재의 증명을 하는 것이 불가능하다." Ibid., 56. *필자 주: 강조를 위해 볼드 및 이탤릭으로 임의 표기하였다.

14. "[...] there is an organic ***whole*** between the individual and the collective that cannot be separated like fish and water; this organic part-whole relation is the condition of the theory of individuation." Hui, 194. *필자 주: 강조를 위해 볼드 및 이탤릭으로 임의 표기하였으며, 참고문헌의 번역본이 국내에 출판되지 않아 영문 본문을 유지하였다.

15. "우주적인 가치의 서열로 올려진, 우주공간 속에서 대체된 지구 거주지의 일상성 자체, 우주공간의 초월성 속으로 실재의 위성화, 이것은 형이상학의 종말이고 환상의 종말이며, 공상과학의 종말이고 ***파생실재성***시기의 시작이다." 보드리야르, 201–202. *필자 주: 강조를 위해 볼드 및 이탤릭으로 임의 표기하였다.

16. "[...] cybernetic machines are acquiring a kind of organicity, thus becoming the ***organizing*** inorganic." Hui, 29. *필자 주: 강조를 위해 볼드 및 이탤릭으로 임의 표기하였으며, 참고문헌의 번역본이 국내에 출판되지 않아 영문 본문을 유지하였다.

17. "Organology signifies a shift from one recursive form (in nature) to another. It is a synthetic thought that not only integrates but also searches for a new epistemology that creates a new loop. Georges Canguilhem was the first, as far as we know, to propose the term general organology in order to rethink the relation between ***organism*** and machine, a rethinking that does not take the machine as the equivalent of the human but rather thinks of the human-machine as an organic whole." Ibid., 25. *필자 주: 강조를 위해 볼드 및 이탤릭으로 임의 표기하였으며, 참고문헌의 번역본이 국내에 출판되지 않아 영문 본문을 유지하였다.

18. "Cosmotechnics means primarily the unification of moral and cosmic order through technical activities; this ***unification*** is a reattachment of the figure to the ground, but it is not a return to

metaphysics of the one and the all." Ibid., 29. *필자 주: 강조를 위해 볼드 및 이탤릭으로 임의 표기하였으며, 참고문헌의 번역본이 국내에 출판되지 않아 영문 본문을 유지하였다.

김현정

「자유롭게, 이리저리, 슬슬」

낯선 길을 나선 나는 불안한 마음으로 새벽부터 서두르는 바람에 너무 일찍 양덕원에 도착해버렸다. 그렇게 나는 마중을 나오기로 한 행복공장 스태프를 기다렸다. 소박하고 조용한 동네를 거닐며 나는 이방인이 된 것 같았다.

최근 행복공장 뉴스 취재 영상을 본 것이 생각났다. 나는 앞으로 감옥과 같은 곳에서 지내야 한다는 사실을 깨닫고는 충격에 빠졌다. 그저 홀로 세상과 잠시 차단되어 하루를 보내고 그 순간 자연스럽게 느끼는 감각, 감성 등에 대한 에세이를 작성하면 된다고 생각했기 때문이다.

하지만 행복공장에 도착하여 내가 머무는 방이 폐문된 이후에도 방송자료를 통해 느꼈던 공포, 두려움은 느낄 수 없었다. 끼니때마다 감옥처럼 방문 아래에 뚫린 사각형 문을 통하여 배식을 받았다. 이러한 방식은 낯설고 불편하기보다 오히려 새롭고 흥미롭게 느껴졌다. 스마트폰조차 없는 상태에서 내가 할 수 있는 일이라고는 한동안 읽지 못했던 책을 집중해서 읽고, 기도하고, 편지를 쓰고, 낮잠을 자는 것 정도였다. 그럼에도 불구하고 방 안에 뚫린 창으로 겨울 풍경을 내내 볼 수 있다는 점은 내게 커다란 위안이 되었다.

나는 낮잠을 자면서 무의식과 만나게 되었던 것 같다. 미처 깔끔하게 마무리되지 못했다고 생각했던 과거의 관계에 대한 깨달음이 섬광처럼 나의 마음 깊은 곳으로, 예고도 없이 찾아왔다. 왜 그럴 수밖에 없었는지, 그 당시에는 도저히 풀리지 않던 숙제처럼 무거웠던 문제들이 예상치 못한 순간에 엉켰던 실타래가 풀리듯 해결되기 시작했다. 이내 나의 몸은 가벼워졌고 마음은 후련해졌다.

행복공장 1.5평의 방은 전혀 좁지 않았다. 평소에 내가

가지고 살아가는 많은 물건에 대해 생각했다. 살아가면서 무엇이 그리 많이 필요한지. 잠시라도 불편해지는 상황을 견디지 못하는 나의 탓이 아닐까? 최소한의 공간, 꼭 필요한 만큼의 식사, 읽을거리, 창밖으로 보이는 풍경, 건강한 육신과 영혼만 있어도 과연 만족하며 살아갈 수 있을지 자문해보았다.

나는 황차를 끊임없이 내려 마셨다. 한 모금 마실 때마다 몸 전체가 따스해졌다. 차를 마시면서 고요한 공간에서 유일한 배경음악이 되어준, 차를 내리는 소리에 집중했다. 또르르, 마치 시냇물이 흐르듯, 자연의 소리가 들렸다. 참으로 신비한 경험이었다.

이 방에서 나는 우리가 살아가는 도시와 일상에서 들리지 않는 소리를 들을 수 있었다. 드디어 내면의 소리에 귀 기울일 수 있게 된 것이다. 꽤 오랜 시간 동안 나는 나의 감정에 충실하지도, 살뜰하지도 못했다. 나는 나 자신을 돌보지 않았다. 하지만 이곳에서는 이 모든 것이 의식의 흐름을 따라 자연스럽게 이루어지고 있었다. 나는 이러한 순간을 간절히 소망해왔는지도 모른다.

이곳을 떠나 일상으로 다시 돌아간다고 해도, 나는 그런 환경을 어떻게 만들 수 있는지에 관해 최소한의 아이디어를 배웠다고 믿는다. 내 삶 자체가 스스로 가두고 또 벗어나고 싶어했던 감옥이었던 것은 아닌지, 내 행동에 대한 정당성을 부여하기 위해 내 삶이 다른 이들을 비난하는 공간이 되지는 않았는지 태어나서 처음으로 고민해 보았던 이 시간을 나는 기억할 것이다.

*

2014년 세월호 사건[1]을 기점으로 한국 사회는 이제껏 겪지 못한 새로운 '디지털 연대'의 시대를 목격했다. 나 또한 이를 목도했지만, 사건에 대한 서로의 견해가 다르다는 이유로 논쟁을 벌이다가 관계를 절연한 경우도 보았다. 이러한 과정을 지켜보면서, 나는 이러한 현상에 휩쓸리지 않은 채 적절한 거리를 유지하고 싶었던 것 같다.

사건이 일어나기 전, 나는 냉철한 판단력 없이 미디어를 믿어 왔다. 하지만, 그러한 미디어는 지속적인 연대로 공동체를 형성하는 다양한 디지털 플랫폼보다 여론에 큰 영향을 미치지 않는 듯했다. 사회 변혁을 야기하는 강력한 힘이 위에서 아래로 강요된 것이 아니라, 바닥에서부터 시작된 것이다. 나는 이러한 현상이 디지털 플랫폼을 통해 대중이 연대감을 형성했기에 가능했다는 점을 강조하고 싶었다. 연대감과 같은 감정이나 정서를 설명하는 것은 어려운 일이지만, '정동'이라는 함축적인 개념으로 표현할 수는 있을 것이다.

이러한 생각에서 시작하여 2018년, 나는 백남준 아트센터에서 《웅얼거리고 일렁거리는》 전시를 기획했다. 나는 이 전시가 당시 불꽃처럼, 용광로처럼 '웅얼거리고 일렁였던' 다양한 목소리에 귀 기울이는 연대의 장이 되기 바랐다. 《웅얼거리고 일렁거리는》은 디지털 네트워크 환경에서 공동의 행동을 이끌어내고, 예상치 못한 사회정치적 변화를 가져온 당시의 다양한 감정을 주제로 기획되었다. 불안하고 위태로운 감정의 흐름과 감각을 동시대 미술로 전환한 이 전시는 총 13팀의 작가 및 그룹으로 구성되었다.[2]

*

> 잠재성은 (…) 그 무언가가 무언가로 현실화되어 변화하기 바로 직전에 머무는 곳입니다. 영구히 그래 왔고, 앞으로도 영원히 머물 곳이죠. (…) 가능성은 상상만 이용하면 만들 수 있습니다. 반대로 잠재성은 만들어질 수 없습니다. 오직 그 발생 가능성만을 만들 수 있죠. 잠재성과 관련해서 보장된 것, 확실한 것은 그 무엇도 없으며, 계산될 수도 없습니다. 잠재성은 확률이 아니라 우연의 문제입니다. 필요한 유일한 것은, 무언가가 발생하는 것입니다.[3]

마텐 스팽베르크의 관점에서 1인 퍼포먼스로 간주될 수 있는 행복공장에서의 24시간을 생각해보면, 나는 내 몸 안의 우연적인 잠재성에 집중했던 것 같다.[4] 나는 나의 의문과 호기심 모두를 탐구하고 싶었다. 그간 인식하지 못했던 신체와 영혼의 상태를 발견할 수 있을지, 그리고 계산과 이성적 판단을 배제한 채 나 자신을 내려놓을 수 있을지 궁금했다. 어쩌면 그 어떤 목적도 갖지 말았어야 했던 것 같다.

내 방은 마치 동굴과 같아서 더 큰 세상, 그리고 나를 따라다니는 불운, 마치 한나 아렌트의 『발터 벤야민: 1892~1940』 에세이에 등장하는 '작은 꼽추'로부터 벗어날 수 있었다. 아렌트는 이 허구의 인물을 불운으로 점철된 벤야민 삶의 모티브로 보았다. 그는 문학 속 정치 싸움에서 벤야민이 어떻게 대처했는지 아래와 같이 설명했다.

> 벤야민은 사정을 알지 못했다. 그는 그런 일들을 어떻게 다룰지 전혀 알지 못했으며, 그런 사람들과 전혀 어울릴 수 없었다. 때로는 늑대들처럼 사방에서 몰려오는 외부 생활의 역경

> 들이 (…) 이미 그에게 세상 물정에 대한 통찰을 얼마간 제공했음에도 불구하고 말이다. 여하간 발 디딜 어떤 확고한 기반을 얻기 위해 적응하고 협조하려고 노력할 때마다, 일은 반드시 잘못되었다.[5]

*

다시 일상으로 돌아온 지금, 나는 안산 경기도미술관에서 세월호 참사 7주기 추념 전시를 준비하고 있다. 미술관 바로 앞 주차장은 사건 당시 합동분향소로 사용되었다.[6]

코로나 팬데믹과 더불어 세월호 사건을 다시 생각해보며 나는 재난 속에서의, 그리고 위로가 필요한 사람들을 위한 예술의 역할에 대해 고민한다. 전시 《웅얼거리고 일렁거리는》은 디지털 플랫폼을 다양한 사건이 발생하면서도 그 어떤 결론도 내려지지 않는 열린 포럼으로 해석했다. 3년이 지난 지금, 세월호 참사 7주기 추념전이 또 다른 공공의 공간, 재난에 의해 잃어버린 영혼을 잊지 않고 기억하는 공간을 만들어낼 수 있기를 바란다.

1. 안산 단원고등학교 학생 325명을 포함해 476명의 승객을 태우고 인천을 출발해 제주도로 향하던 세월호는 2014년 4월 16일 전남 진도군 앞바다에서 급변침을 하며 침몰했다. 구조를 위해 해경이 도착했을 때, "가만히 있으라"는 방송을 했던 선원들이 승객들을 버리고 가장 먼저 탈출했다. 배가 침몰한 이후 구조자는 단 한 명도 없었다. 사고의 원인과 진상규명에 대한 의문은 여전히 남아 있다. 더욱 자세한 정보는 다음 백과사전에서 찾아볼 수 있다. "세월호", 다음 백과, 2021년 4월 1일, https://100.daum.net/encyclopedia/view/47XXXXXXXXX6.

2. 이 전시에 참여한 13명(팀)은 이윤정과 권혜원을 포함하여 70~80년대 생이 주를 이룬다. 특히 해외에서 주목받고 있는 작가들이 참가해 눈길을 끌었다. 해외 작가 에드 앳킨스, 세실 에반스는 당시 국내 미술 저널에서 선정한 동시대 미술가 45인에 이름을 올렸다. 또한 로잘린 나샤시비는 2017년 터너상 후보, 이그나스 크룽레비시우스는 2010년 독일 백남준 상 후보로 이름을 올린 바 있다. 국내 작가 중에서는 함양아와 홍민키의 신작이 소개되었다.

3. Mårten Spångberg, "Post-dance, An Advocacy," in *Post-Dance*, eds. Danjel Andersson, Mette Edvardsen, Mårten Spångberg (Stockholm: MDT, 2017), 379–80.

4. 스팽베르크의 글을 실은 『불가능한 춤』은 오늘날 춤과 무용의 자리를 다시 새롭게 살피는 책이다. 수년간 다원예술 축제를 기획하고 플랫폼을 구축해 온 공연예술 기획자 김성희가 현장에서 작품과 이론을 두루 발표하며 동시대 예술의 한계를 넓혀 나간 여러 무용가와 안무가를 초대하여 춤의 활로를 찾는다. 이들은 무대 위에서, 무대 뒤에서, 무대 밖에서 쓴 글을 통해 지난 성과와 한계를 돌아보며 안무, 관객, 무대, 신체, 언어 등 무용의 기반으로 여겨져 왔던 개념을 새로운 관점과 태도로 다룬다. 마텐 스팽베르크 외, 『불가능한 춤』 (서울: 워크룸프레스, 2020).

5. Hannah Arendt, "Walter Benjamin: 1892–1940," in *Men in Dark Times* (New York: Harcourt, Brace & World, Inc., 1955), 162. 아렌트의 벤야민 전기는 본래 1968년 10월 19일 「뉴요커」에 게재되었다. 이 글은 아렌트가 벤야민의 에세이와 글을 묶어 편집한 『Illuminations』 의 소개글로도 사용되었다.

6. 합동분향소는 세월호 참사 13일 만인 2014년 4월 29일에 세워졌다. 2018년 4월에 폐쇄하기까지 그동안 합동분향소에 다녀간 추모객은 72만 8천 323 명에 이른다. 안산시는 화랑유원지 내 부지를 선정, 영구 추모공원 조성을 계획하고 있다. 이를 위해 시는 지역 주민, 세월호 가족, 전문가 등이 참여하는 '50인 위원회'를 구성하여, 의견을 충분히 수렴해 세부 건립계획을 마련하겠다고 설명했다. 더욱 자세한 정보는 2018년 4월 7일 자 문화일보 "세월호 추모공간 정부합동분향소 4년 만에 문 닫는다" 기사에서 찾아볼 수 있다. 『문화일보』, 2018년 4월 7일, http://www.munhwa.com/news/view.html?no=20180407MW104650908900.

이민경

「파열」

0

‘깨달음’을 얻었다는 한 수감자의 이야기가 기억난다. 그는 결백했지만 장기형을 선고받은 사람이었다. 처음의 충격을 다잡고, 그는 이를 곧 명상의 기회로 삼았다. 결연하고 끊임없는 노력으로 그는 평온해졌고, 자신감과 기쁨을 찾게 되었다. 복역 기간이 끝나갈 무렵, 그는 거의 성자처럼 보였다.

출소일 직전, 그의 석방은 무슨 이유인지 거부되었으며, 형량은 무기한 연장되었다. 그의 평정심과 더불어 성자다운 모습 역시 사라지고 없었다. 그는 완전히 붕괴되었다. 그런데 어느 시점에서인가 무슨 일이 그에게 일어났고, 그는 다시 한번 성자로 거듭났다. 이후 그 면모를 다시는 잃지 않았다고 한다.

이 이야기는 실화로 알고 있는데, 나는 그에게 무슨 일이 일어났던 것일지 궁금해하곤 했다. 이번 ‘감옥’에서의 하루에 초대되면서, 나도 그가 겪은 깨달음의 경험을 조금이나마 얻게 되길 기대했다.

00

이 감옥에서 나는 실제로 갇혀 있지 않았다. 행복공장이 작은 동전을 이용하면 안쪽에서도 문을 열 수 있다는 점을 (비상시에 대비하여) 미리 알려주었을 때, 나는 이미 식사 투입구를 통해 이곳에서 편히 나갈 수 있음을 알아낸 상태였다. 언제든지 방에서 나갈 수 있다는 걸 알게 되자, 나는 편안히 이 갇힌

상태에서의 모의 실험을 즐길 수 있었다.

행복공장의 환경은 매우 쾌적했고, 24시간은 꽤나 짧을 듯했다. 나는 이 시간을 명상이나 수면과 같이 내게 당연한 활동으로 채우지 않기로 결심했다. 내 정신이 다른 어딘가로 가거나 무의식으로 빠져들지 않기를 바랐다. 마치 인류학자처럼, 나는 내게 어떤 정신적, 감정적 상태가 생겨나는지에 주의를 기울였다. 내 정신을 면밀히 따라가며, 다른 것에 주의를 뺏기지 않으려 노력했다.

000

오슬로에서 진행했던 프로젝트가 떠올랐다. 우리는 그걸 〈공원 벤치 프로젝트(A Park Bench Project)〉[1]라고 불렀다. 깨달음을 얻게 된 이후 2년간 공원 벤치에서 시간을 보내며 더 없는 행복을 느꼈다는 에크하르트 톨레의 이야기로부터 직접적인 영감을 받은 것이었다.[2]

친구 몬세라트[3]와 나는 톨레의 상태를 모방해보려 했다. 매일 우리는 극장 근처 공원 벤치에 앉아 아무것도 하지 않는 것을 연습했다. 공연 날 우리는 극장의 큰 홀 한가운데에 비어 있는 벤치를 몇 개 놓은 다음, 그곳에 앉아 관객들을 '특별히 뭔가 하지 않기'에 동참하도록 하였다. 나는 일상생활에서 하듯 항시 움직인 한편, 몬세라트는 꼼짝 않고 앉아 있었다. 청중들은 벤치나 공간 곳곳에 앉아 매우 다양한 종류의 '아무것도 하지 않기'를 함께했다. 여러 사람들이 같이 어울리는 쾌활한 모임이었다.

공원 벤치에 앉아 몇 년이나 행복해했던 톨레의 모습을 상상할 때, 나는 그가 특별히 아무것도 하지 않는, 심지어 명상조차 하지 않는 모습을 떠올린다. 지두 크리슈나무르티는 그의 책에서 명상에 대해 자주 이야기했는데, 그가 늘 강조한 건 명상이란 하는 것이 아니라 일어나는 것이라는 점이었다.[4] (명상이 당신에게 '일어나지' 않는다면 꽤나 답답한 일이다.)

명상은 보통 내게 '일어나지' 않았기 때문에 나는 20여 년간 배우고 연습하기를 불규칙적으로 반복했다. 대부분 내가 노력하며 시간을 보냈고, 명상은 간간이 저절로 일어나기도 했다.

0000

3개월 명상 수행 중에 말 그대로 아무것도 하지 않아 보려 한 적이 한 번 있다. 저녁 시간 내내 침대에 누워 눈을 뜨고 있었다. 나는 자세를 바꾸거나 눈을 깜빡이는 일 등 뭔가를 하지 않을 수가 없다는 걸 아주 재빨리 깨달았다. 내가 끊임없이 무언가를 하도록 만든 것은 불편, 또는 불교 용어로 '고(苦)'였다.

그 수행 기간이 끝나가던 어느 날 아침, 잠에서 깨면서 갑작스레 내 정신은 움직이지 않는 상태에 들어갔다. 의식이 온전히 깨어 있었음에도 그 어떤 생각, 감정, 움직임도 없었다. 그 경험에 대한 묘사도 지나고 나서 돌이켜 생각했을 때야 가능했다. 내 정신은 '정상'으로 돌아오기 전까지 한동안 그 상태에 멈춰 있었다.

나는 의식이 정신으로부터 독립적이라는 가설, 혹은 특

정한 신체와 정신 너머에 존재하는 의식이라는 가설에 관해 여러 차례 듣고 읽어 왔다.[5] 그때 나는 의식의 형이상학과 정신의 본질에 대해 유추해 볼 수 있는 하나의 경험적인 데이터를 직접 얻은 셈이었다.

그 이후 이 경험은 반복되지 않았다.

000

행복공장은 감옥에서의 경험을 할 수 있다고 홍보하긴 했지만, 조금 찾아보고 나니 이곳의 24시간 프로그램이 '무문관(無門關)'의 짧은 버전이라는 사실을 알게 되었다. 무문관은 본래 한국을 비롯한 여러 나라에서 이루어져 온 불교 수행인데, 수행자들은 방이나 집에 들어가 문을 잠그고 몇 달 이상이 될 수도 있는 수행 기간 동안 나오지 않는다. 행복공장이 독방 감옥만큼이나 명상처를 전유했다는 점이 명확해졌다. 명상과 안거에 관한 경험자인 나 또한 깜박 속인 이 감옥과 명상처 사이의 혼돈 가능성은 이 두 곳의 목적과 특성에 대해 재차 생각해보지 않을 수 없게 했다.

이들의 공통적이고 핵심적인 특징은 정신적 파열을 촉진한다는 점이라고 하겠다. 두 군데 다 감각적 자극과 사회적 접촉을 박탈하여 자신의 정신 외에 남는 자극이 거의 없게 한다. 감각적 자극은 우리의 정신세계를 위한 원재료 혹은 구성요소로서 기능하며, 이미지와 개념, 시간과 서사, 현상의 해석, 정체성 등의 생성을 가능하게 한다. 독방 감금과 명상 수행이 이들을 모두 없애 버리고 나면, 사람들은 아마 기억, 현

실, 그리고 정체성의 인식에 있어 변화를 겪게 될 것이다. 그들 주변 세계의 견고함이나 구체성에 대해서도 더 이상 확신하지 못하게 될 것이며, 이로 인해 자아 정체성이 궁극적으로는 해체되거나 소멸에 이를 수도 있다.

평범한 인간에게 이러한 파열은 고통스러운 것이며, 광기나 죽음에까지 이르게 하는 충격이 될 수 있다. 감옥이나 명상 수행처의 관점에서는 목표가 달성된 것이리라.

00

만약 명상 수행이 그런 파열(break)을 가능하게 한다면, 이는 어떻게 인간의 붕괴(breakdown)가 아닌 돌파(breakthrough)를 야기하는 것일까? 최근 몇 년간의 대중적 이해와는 다른 명상 수행 경험에 관한 부정적이고 충격적인 보고도 존재한다. 나는 수행이나 수도원 생활 중 정신 상태가 악화된 세 사람을 개인적으로 알고 있다. 물론, 더욱 행복한 상태가 되어 수행처를 떠난 이들도 300명 정도는 알 것이다. 그렇지만 정신은 부정적인 경향도 가득 안고 있다. 그런 지뢰밭을 건너는 건 쉬운 일이 아니다.

명상에서 중요한 요소는 사람들이 부정적이고 해로운 생각 및 감정에 빠져들지 않도록 하는 동시에, 긍정적이고 너그러운 생각과 감정을 키워나가는 데 있다. 이는 감옥의 독방 감금에서는 제공해주지 않는 경험이다. 비유하자면, 장기적인 단식은 안전하게 할 경우 건강에 큰 도움이 되지만, 그렇지 않을 경우 심각한 위험이 된다.

앞서 깨달음을 얻은 죄수를 언급한 이유는 그를 모델로 삼기 위해서가 아니다. 그는 결국 난관을 돌파했지만, 그 과정에서는 거의 붕괴될 뻔했다. 심지어 엄청난 고행을 통해 깨달은 부처조차도 다른 이들에게는 이를 따를 것을 권하지 않았다. 확실하지 않다면, 좀 더 안전하고 이미 입증된 길을 걷는 편이 나을 것이다: 부드럽고 다정하게 파열을 향해 나아가기. 즐겁게, 즐겁게.

0

유년시절. 내게는 좋은 시절이었다. 돈을 벌어야 할 필요도, 집이나 가족, 경력 등 그 무엇도 관리할 필요도 없었다. 너무도 단순했고, 매일이 휴일이었다. 내가 한 것은 그저 먹고, 놀고, 엄마 말씀 잘 듣고, 자라는 것뿐이었다. 그때를 돌이켜보면, 그 단조로움이 일종의 충격으로 느껴진다.

야외에서 긴 시간을 뛰어논 후, 작은 기쁨과 함께 텅 비게 되는 그 강렬한 느낌을 기억한다. 하늘과 구름도 더욱 빛나던 걸 기억한다. 그 느낌은 광대하고 가벼웠다. 광대하고도 가볍다는 것 — 내게 있어 명상을 가장 잘 묘사하는 표현이다.

행복공장에서 나오던 날 아침, 잠겨 있던 문이 다시 열리기 몇 시간 전, 내가 그 어떤 깨달음도 얻지 못할 것이라는 게 명확해졌다. 모든 긴장과 기대, 기다림과 관찰을 내려놓았고, 나는 곧 편안해졌다. 이전 참가자들이 남기고 간 재미있고 중요한 (혹은 중요하지 않은) 글귀나 그림을 보며 시간을 죽여도 상관없었다. 나도 하나 남기고 왔다. 내 자신이 뭐든

하도록 내버려두었다. 그러자 마치 어린시절에 그랬듯이 즐겁고 가벼워졌다. 붕괴로든 돌파로든 파열은 내게 일어나지 않았다. 이번에는.

1. 〈공원 벤치 프로젝트〉는 2009년 오슬로 단센스 후스에서 스윗엔텐더 콜레보레이션스와 미아 하비브가 개최한 〈리빙 하우스〉 중 일부였다.

2. Eckhart Tolle, *The Power of Now: A Guide to Spiritual Enlightenment* (Vancouver: Namaste Publishing, 1997) 참조.

3. 멕시코 무용가 몬세라트 파요.

4. J. Krishnamurti, *Krishnamurti's Journal* (New York: HarperCollins, 1982) 참조.

5. 불교를 포함한, 인더스 문명에서 발생된 종교들 다수에서 주장하는 이론이다.

타일러 코번은 뉴욕 기반 예술가 및 작가로서 파리 퐁피두센터, 뉴욕 휘트니미술관, 베르겐 쿤스트할, 쿤스트할레 빈, 런던 헤이워드 갤러리, 홍콩 파라사이트, 서울 아트선재센터 등에서 작업을 선보였다. 그는 『I'm that angel』(2012), 『Robots Building Robots』(글래스고 현대미술센터, 2013), 『Richard Roe』(스턴버그 프레스, 2019)의 저자이다. 또한, 이플럭스, 프리즈, 아트리뷰, DIS, 무스, LEAP, 리좀 등의 매거진에 기고한 바 있다.

김경묵은 극영화와 다큐멘터리, 비디오아트, 영상설치 등 다양한 형식과 매체를 오가며 작업해온 영상작가이다. 2004년 단편 다큐멘터리 〈나와 인형놀이〉로 데뷔하여 2005년 〈얼굴 없는 것들〉, 2011년 〈줄탁동시〉, 2014년 〈이것이 우리의 끝이다〉 등 다수의 영화를 제작했다. 이 작품들은 베니스영화제, 로테르담영화제, 런던영화제, 밴쿠버영화제, 시드니영화제, 부에노스아이레스영화제, 홍콩영화제 등 세계 유수의 영화제와 MoMA, New Museum, 일민미술관, 아르코미술관 등에서 상영 및 전시되었으며 다수의 상을 수상했다.

유지원은 서울을 기반으로 활동하는 큐레이터, 비평가, 통번역가이다. 관심경제와 플랫폼 자본주의의 교차점에 놓인 노동, 대중 매체와 시각 문화에서의 젠더 재현, 큐레토리얼 실천에서의 유물주의적 접근을 중점적으로 탐구하고 있다. 대표 전시로는 《유어서치, 내 손 안의 리서치 서비스》(공동기획, 두산갤러리 서울, 2018), 《(Not) Your Typical Narcissist》(온라인, 2019–진행 중), 《그래비티 샤워》(대한극

장, N/A, 2020–2021) 등이 있다. 2019년부터 2021년까지 제11회 서울미디어시티비엔날레 어시스턴트 큐레이터로 근무하였다.

이우창은 서울대학교 영문과 박사과정에서 18세기 영국소설 및 지성사를 공부하고 있으며, 새뮤얼 리처드슨의 소설과 영국의 "초기 여성주의" 담론에 관해 박사논문을 준비하고 있다. 오늘날 한국의 담론 및 논쟁에 관해서도 다양한 글을 쓴다. 「헬조선 담론의 기원」(2016), 「'서구 근대'의 위기와 한국 동아시아 담론의 기이한 여정」(2017), "The Politics and Sub-Politics of Mad Cow Disease in South Korea" (공저, 2022) 등의 학술논문을 썼으며, 2020년 리처드 왓모어의 『지성사란 무엇인가?』를 한국어로 번역했다.

김선진은 대전에서 활동하는 아티스트 및 작가이다. 서울대학교 디자인학부 시각디자인과를 졸업하였으며, 그간 〈#FriendlyStrangers〉(광주디자인비엔날레, 2017), 라이브 팟캐스트 퍼포먼스 〈테이크투〉(비둘기 오디오 & 비디오 페스티벌, 2017), 〈고홈솔져 프로젝트〉(블로그, 2011) 등을 진행했다.

정재연은 한국예술종합학교 조형예술과를 졸업하고, 영국 첼시예술대학원에서 순수미술로 석사학위를 받았다. 2012년까지 런던에서 작업하였으며, 이후 귀국하여 서울에서 활동하고 있다. 그는 최근 서울에 《로스트 코너》(아트스페이스 그로브, 2018)와 《로스트 코너_메모리 아카이브》(SeMA

창고, 2019) 등 두 차례 개인전을 선보였으며, 영국을 비롯해 미국, 독일, 오스트리아, 대만, 일본에서 다수의 기획전과 레지던시 프로그램에 참여했다. 그의 작업은 장소 특정적 설치와 영상을 결합하며, 기억, 역사, 집단 정체성, 그리고 건축에 관한 이슈에 초점을 맞추고 있다. 현재 남편 러셀 메이슨과 함께 서울에 거주 중이다.

러셀 메이슨은 1976년 영국 랭커셔주 블랙번에서 출생했다. 그는 역사를 전공한 후 영어 교사가 되었으며, 지난 25년간 어학원 및 대학에서 외국인 학생들에게 영어를 가르쳐 왔다. 그는 10년 전 런던에서 부인 정재연을 만나 4년 뒤 한국으로 이주하였다. 메이슨은 현재 고려대학교에서 1학년 학부생 대상 학술 영어 교과목을 담당하고 있다.

여인영은 서울에 거주하는 아티스트이다. 그의 작업은 텍스트, 드로잉 및 설치를 예술적으로 구체화하는 것부터 그의 주요 연구 분야인 젠더, 인공지능 및 도시화에 대한 학제간 전시기획에 이르기까지 다양하다. 그는 패턴, 숫자, 인간 '마음'의 논리적 구조에 기반을 둔 차원, 그리고 다차원적 시공간에서의 우연을 탐구한다. 이러한 호기심은 주기적 '관계'에 초점을 맞춘 미시적 내러티브 관련 연구에 기인한다. 여인영은 한국, 독일, 동남아시아를 포함한 여러 지역에서 프로젝트, 전시, 레지던시, 토크, 워크숍 등을 기획하고 참여했다.

김현정은 변화하는 미디어 환경에 따른 디지털 사회의 현상, 특히 사람들의 소통 방식에 관심을 두고 있는 큐레이터

이다. 백남준아트센터의 《웅얼거리고 일렁거리는》(2018), 《슈퍼전파-미디어바이러스》(2015)를 포함하여 다수의 전시를 기획하였다. 또한, 광주비엔날레, 부산비엔날레, 경기창작센터 등 다양한 전시 및 프로젝트에 참여했다. 그는 최근 2021년 11월 안산 경기도미술관에서의 중견 작가 3인전을 준비한 바 있다. 전시뿐만 아니라 현대미술 아카데미, 문화자원봉사 교육프로그램 기획을 통하여 예술을 공유하는 여러 방식을 끊임없이 고민하고 있다.

이민경은 무용가, 공연예술가로서 뉴질랜드와 유럽을 거쳐 현재 한국에서 활동 중이다. 경험으로서의 춤, 설득의 과정과 확신의 심리적 상태, 현 시대에 예술가로 살아가는 조건에 관한 작업들을 해왔다. 공연의 형식적 실험에 관심을 갖고 실시간 실험을 포함하는 무대극, 관객이 실질적 공연자로 참여하여 성립시키는 공연게임, 선언으로서의 공연 등을 창조하며 공연 형식의 확장을 추구했다. 국제 예술가 네트워크인 스윗엔텐더 콜레보레이션스의 공동 창립 멤버이자 아카데미 슐로스 솔리튜드 펠로우, 댄스웹 장학생, 국립현대미술관 창동레지던시 입주작가로 활동하였다. 주요 작품으로 〈게리를 공산주의자로 전향시키는 데 얼마나 걸리나〉, 〈그는 무대에서 춤을 추었나〉, 〈일명, 중국 오페라〉, 〈봄의 제전 (2013)〉, 〈예술이어야 한다면〉, 〈저드슨 드라마(취소선)〉, 〈삼물기(三物記)〉 등이 있다.